ROM
BATHS
IN BRITAIN

ABOUT THE AUTHOR

Ian D. Rotherham is Professor of Environmental Geography and Reader in Tourism & Environmental Change at Sheffield Hallam University. He is a historian, ecologist and environmental geographer and has written over 400 articles, papers, books and book chapters. He also writes and broadcasts on history and environmental issues for newspapers, radio and television, including the BBC History Programme.

ROMAN BATHS IN BRITAIN

IAN D. ROTHERHAM

AMBERLEY

First published 2012

Amberley Publishing
The Hill, Stroud
Gloucestershire, GL5 4EP

www.amberleybooks.com

British Library Cataloguing in Publication Data.
A catalogue record for this book is available from the British Library.

ISBN 978 1 4456 0657 6

Typeset in 10pt on 12pt Sabon.
Typesetting and Origination by Amberley Publishing.
Printed in the UK.

CONTENTS

PREFACE

Focusing on Britain and the impacts of Roman occupation on the British, this volume introduces the idea and culture of baths and bathing that grew during Roman times. This was the pinnacle of sophisticated leisure and of cleanliness and central to Roman society. With the fall of Rome, it would be a thousand years before anything approaching the technology and importance developed anywhere in Europe. After the collapse of the Roman Empire, even the most high-ranking people in European society were distinctly grubby and smelly! Yet Roman baths and bathing culture influenced the spas and baths that grew out of the medieval period. Even the physical structures, albeit as ruins, remained in cities such as Bath in England and Caerleon in Wales. Today, where significant structures remain as in Leicester city centre, Caerleon, and especially Bath, they are once again great visitor attractions. Bath and its restored bathhouses is perhaps the most famous of these sites, and it also boasts the most intact Roman system remaining in Europe.

The book explores the importance of water to the Romans, and the idea of cleanliness to their physical and mental well-being. We examine the role of baths and bathing in many facets of Roman life, which reached levels of sophistication, and sometimes excess, which have perhaps never been exceeded since. Finally, we find out what the Roman traditions and constructions have left as heritage and archaeology today and where we can go to find out more about the way of life and the unique and fascinating history of baths and bathing. This was something deeply embedded in Roman culture and became a facet of Roman, or in Britain 'Romanised', life that separated the civilised from the heathens. The Roman would bathe before his main meal and the wealthy had their own bathrooms where they could be washed, oiled, scraped and massaged by their household slaves. However, an important development across the Empire, from Rome itself to the far-flung provinces, was the public access to great bathhouses. Successive Consuls and Emperors provided the public with magnificent *thermae*; palaces dedicated to bathing and associated activities. These were places where the Romans gathered, as they also did at the public latrines, to chat, to gossip and to exchange news and views. Some facilities offered mixed nude bathing and more, and were viewed with suspicion and disapproval by the more conservative and reputation-conscious citizens. Men generally wore leather trunks and the women a brief loin-cloth.

The book focuses on examples from across Britain but especially from the city whose name is synonymous with Roman bathing – Bath. It is richly illustrated with images, both prints and photographs, from the past. All images are from the author's personal collection unless otherwise stated. The modern photographs are courtesy of Bath & North East Somerset Council.

Spas, healing baths and also mineral waters are enjoying a revival during the late twentieth and early twenty-first centuries, but their origins go back to the Romano-British and beyond. However, the direct links to the past of many now old spas are often tenuous. Local rumours and myths frequently relate a spa or a spring to ancient Roman usage, even when there is no evidence whatsoever for such a link. Many such sites probably extend back to Georgian or early Victorian times but no further. Yet there undoubtedly exist the remains of numerous genuinely Romano-British bathhouse sites still to be discovered in lost villas, farmhouses and perhaps even small forts. Some known sites in Britain are described here and many of these are open to visitors.

1

THE ROMANS, WATER & BATHING

The Romans were the first people to build baths, bathhouses, and particularly public baths. They were also the first to place a sense of social occasion on bathing and taking the waters, and like the Celts before them they linked special sites to appropriate deities. For the Romans, the significant mineral springs like Aquae Sulis at Bath, Aquae Arnemetiae at Buxton, and perhaps lesser sites at Droitwich and Ilkley were important locations. The great bathhouses at these special sites would have been significant in the regional and national social round. Across the wider countryside, the greater farms and villas also had baths and bathhouses, and the provision at military centres such as Caerleon in South Wales, and Chester in north-west England were large, luxurious installations. With the import of Roman baths to Britain, it was not just the buildings which were important but the culture of bathing too. Furthermore, when the Romans left, the buildings crumbled and the social significance of communal bathing was lost.

Just as in Rome itself, the great bathhouses and spas provided music, drama, poetry, business and commerce, medicine, personal grooming, and a chance to catch up and to gossip. The baths would be a focus for local traders and others: barbers, masseurs, physicians, food-vendors, wine-sellers, musicians, pimps, procurers and prostitutes. Here, away from the rigours of the provincial front line, soldiers could relax and recuperate, and local citizens could mingle and enjoy their leisure. In this heady mix of water, heat, money and commerce, they were people prepared to take your money and to provide whatever you needed or wanted. Amongst other things, these great bathhouses were the places to see and to be seen.

We must remember too that Romano-British Britain was a largely slave-based economy, and the bathhouses were no exception to this. The baths at Aquae Sulis or at Aquae Arnemetiae would have depended to a great extent on slave-labour for their day-to-day working. Comparisons have been drawn between the economic slavery that delivered the spa experiences in Bath in the seventeenth and eighteenth centuries, and diarists such as Celia Fiennes certainly suggested that this was little different from the Roman system. Each society was able to create and deliver an efficient and splendid service for the upper echelons that made up their patrons. A notable change might have been the absence in the spas of eighteenth century Bath, of the young boy attendants that the older male Romans were so keen on. Even so, it was suggested that the waters of Bath were not merely enjoyed for their curative powers. Ned Ward, a satirist who wrote *A Step to Bath*, was perhaps exaggerating, but only a little:

> Here is performed all the wanton dalliance imaginable; celebrated beauties, panting breasts and curious shapes, almost exposed to public view; languishing eyes, darting killing glances, tempting amorous postures, attended by soft music, enough to provoke a vestal to forbidden pleasure, captivate a saint and charm a Jove. The vigorous sparks present the ladies with several antick postures, as sailing on their backs, then embracing the element, sink in a rapture and by accidental design thrust an outstretched arm; but where the water concealed, so ought my pen. The spectators in the galleries please their roving fancies with this lady's face, another's eyes, a third's heavy breasts and profound air. In one corner stood an old lecher whose years bespoke him not less than three-score and ten, making love to a young lady not exceeding fourteen.

Water and sources of clean water have always been important to people, and in times past were revered and even worshipped. Springs, wells and spas were considered to be places of special powers and magic, gifts from the gods, and so were revered as special places. Pre-Roman cultures such as the Celts had similar responses to the thermal springs at, for example, Bath. Indeed, this worship of watering places continued after the fall of the Roman Empire, as Christianity largely banned bathing, but miraculous and curative springs were a different matter. Sites such as Walsingham in Norfolk became major places for Christian pilgrimage as a spring was said to emanate from the spot where a local girl had seen the Virgin Mary. The Blessed Virgin had appeared to a local swineherd in AD 1061, and a spring had miraculously erupted from the spot to mark the occasion. The location remains today a major tourism and pilgrimage attraction.

Some of the associations go back long before the Romans arrived in Britain. The warm mineral waters of Bath were already in use before the bathhouses of Aquae Sulis. Supposedly the Celtic King Bladud, the father of the model for Shakespeare's King Lear, developed leprosy and so left his court to become a humble swineherd. However, with an astute piece of observation he noticed that his pigs were cured of skin complaints by wallowing in the mud. He followed them into the swamp and immersed himself in the curative warm mud, and the treatment eventually cured him. George Kersley writing in 1973 suggested that Bladud might have been suffering from some other skin complaint such as scabies and this would make it more amenable to cure. This is the site of the ancient baths today and in legend at least, was the foundation of Bath's long history of curative, health-giving powers. The thermal waters of the area had certainly attracted Celtic interest and reverence to the extent of the location being called Sul, after a Celtic goddess. Aquae Sulis of the Romans was simply an adoption of the earlier dedication, and the special nature of the site was recognised in their double dedication of Sul Minerva to link the Celtic goddess with their own goddess of medicine. Buxton in the north Midlands and Droitwich also may have been Roman spas. The former has extensive Roman remains and may have been a rest centre for legionaries based on the northern frontier. Yet it was Bath itself that was pre-eminent in Britain as a Romano-British spa and bath. A significant Roman town developed on the site and this served an area that was to become extensively developed by the Romans and their *colonia* or settlements for retired soldiers. The climate here was good and would be favourable for rich and wealthy Romans or the Romano-British who had become rich under the Empire. With good villas scattered across the farming lands of the Cotswolds and the proximity to the garrison town of *Glevum* (modern-day Gloucester), this was a location guaranteed to prosper under the Roman occupation.

Before we move onto bathing, it is worth considering the nature of the chemical itself. Water is a compound made up of two the elements, Hydrogen and Oxygen, with one part of the latter to two of the former, to give us the well-known H_2O formula. Yet few people realise what a special and indeed unusual chemical this is; familiarity breeds contempt. A liquid at room temperature, water evaporates to a gas and freezes to a solid. The Hydrogen atom is small, and has a tendency to give away its negatively charged electron, and so develop a positive charge. Oxygen tends to accept electrons, and so it becomes negatively charged. This exchange of electrons basically binds the atoms together as the chemical compound 'water'. But there is more, and it is the charged nature of the water molecule that is responsible. The chemical bonds that form the molecule are strong, but the positive Hydrogen atoms of one molecule are also attracted to the negative Oxygen atom in adjacent water molecules; opposites attract. These so-called 'Hydrogen bonds' have important impacts on the behaviour of water in both its physical manifestations and its chemical ones too. So the charged or 'ionic' character allows water to dissolve substances such as salts which are so important to the 'healing waters' we encounter later in the book. This same character helps water to dissolve certain charged organic chemicals but mean that it fails to do this with other organic substances such as oils and grease. To cleanse the bodies of these substances which are insoluble in water we need to use organic cleansing agents like soaps and oils.

The peculiar nature of its chemical and physical bonding is also responsible for the fact that water, unlike all other liquids, becomes less dense as its temperature approaches freezing point. If, like most substances, water just got denser and so became heavier as it cooled, then for example, ice would not form on top of a pond or lake, but it would freeze from the bottom up. Life as we know it could not have evolved in such an environment, and water is almost unique in this behaviour. Furthermore, even the great oceanic heat-currents that power our climate, taking hot air and water from tropics to poles and *vice versa*, depend on this unique property. Water contracts as it cools until about 4°C, and then it expands and gets lighter until it freezes, and so ice floats on water. Finally, water is hugely abundant in the universe and very important on planet Earth. It is the main component of all living things and so is essential for all life-forms that we know of. Water really is a most remarkable substance, and in baths and bathing is essential for cleansing, and for heating, and for generating the hot humid atmosphere of a steam bath or the cold icy conditions of a cold bath. The water brings renewal and warmth and takes away dirt and waste. It is through manipulating the extreme conditions of water as liquid, gas, condensed clouds of steam, or a freezing cold ice in northern climes, that we produce the conditions of baths, spas and bathing.

Water and its genesis are also closely bound up in ideas of 'Creation' and in myths of catastrophic and destructive floods which occur around the globe and in many different religions. In an instant, water is both a giver of life and a bringer of death and destruction. The Hebrew God in creating the Earth commanded that the water under the sky be gathered into one place – the ocean – and then the world emerged from this infinite primeval ocean to give dry land and the sky. So water is central to life and to humanity and it is the essence of baths and of bathing. We bathe and swim in it, we drink it and absorb it, it washes us and we excrete it too, and through sweat glands it cools us; our bodies are more than 70 per cent water. In actual fact, it is likely that most of our water on Earth actually arrived here long after the planet was formed, since the molten hot volcanic surface of the young planet in the inner heat of the solar system was no place for volatile compounds like H_2O. No, our water arrived in collisions with millions of meteorites, occasionally comets, and other cosmic particles from the cold, icy, outer reaches of the solar system. But that is a different story. When water emerges from underground springs as pure ice-cold liquid or as warm sulphur-rich mineral water, early peoples viewed this occurrence as a special gift from Nature and from their particular gods. Water was a miraculous substance and its occurrence was itself a miracle.

This first chapter sets the scene on how and why baths and bathing developed in Rome and across the Roman Empire. Baths and bathhouses are to be found wherever the Roman civilisation was established and as stated by the pioneering archaeologist Sir Mortimer Wheeler, 'The innumerable public baths of the Roman Empire made an outstanding contribution to the general development of plan and structure.' For the Romans, the baths provided a focus of social, aesthetic, cultural and physical life. Employing a rich array of technologies in designing and operating their baths, many of the sophistications would not be available again for a thousand years after the fall of the Roman Empire. The construction and operation of bathhouses involved the transport and application of materials such as building stone, lead for pipes, bronze for taps and fittings, marble for mosaics, and richly decorated plasterwork form ceilings and walls. The materials and technologies were cleverly applied to provide heating and effective supplies of the necessary water.

We know that baths, initially for men only, existed in Roman life since at least the second century BC. Initially they were places for socializing, for discussing important issues, and for transacting business. They were therefore perhaps not a place for women. Apparently Roman men also socialised and discussed business and politics at the communal latrines. The first baths for men and women are referred to with the neuter word *balneum*, and were private establishments. Presumably they were exclusive and the poorer people did not mingle with the women. Similarly, the poorer citizens had little knowledge or information on business or other important matters of interest to the wealthy patrons of the day. Baths and bathing developed rapidly as the Roman Empire grew. The experimentation and evolution, which took place in design and in operation, is clear from evidence and remains on sites and in modern museums. Bathing was deeply embedded in Roman and Romanised society and culture.

Whilst many people associate the Romans with the invention of formal baths and bathing, ideas of steam baths and similar practices in fact evolved independently in a wide range of different societies from Europe, to the Americas and the Far East. In considering the origins of Roman baths and the culture of bathing the search is most naturally amongst the other Mediterranean and North African civilisations of the time. The novelty of the Roman bath was perhaps in the application of the *hypocaust* with bathing pool suspended on pillars and heated by great boilers. Hypocausts were used by the Greeks, but generally the Roman oyster breeder of Baiae, C. Sergius Orata, is credited with invention of the first such working Roman bath. It is likely that he perfected existing Greek technologies and was the first to have provided effective heating.

It is clear that the value and benefits of immersion of the human body in water have long been recognised. Furthermore, it is evident from history that health, hygiene, and leisure aspects of bathing have changed dramatically with differing and varying cultures over time. However, it is widely recognised that the early heyday of bathing, public and private, was with the Roman Empire, and as this declined, then so did the habit and custom of bathing. As the Empire decayed, then the practice of bathing became restricted to a very few wealthy individuals using private facilities.

From the twelfth century onwards there began a Renaissance in Western Europe that culminated in the Georgian penchant for 'taking the waters' for health reasons. The re-emergence of bathing popularity perhaps owed much to the returning Crusaders who had experienced and enjoyed Turkish Baths in the Middle East and North Africa. By the fourteenth century, Londoners had a choice of at least eighteen bathhouse establishments. Pilgrims would flock to holy wells and bath in their cold mineral waters to seek purification and where necessary, cures for ailments. However, bathing also became increasingly associated with licentiousness and decadence. By the time of the Reformation, attitudes in England changed and saintly miracles, nudity, and indeed contact between water and the human body, were increasingly frowned upon. Warm water in particular was something to be feared and preferably avoided. Washing for hygiene purposes was restricted to hands and face, and in order to minimise offensive odours, a regular change of linen was the accepted protocol. Queen Elizabeth I famously stated that she took a bath once a month – whether she needed it or not. 'Need' was perhaps related more to health reasons than cleanliness.

It was only in the seventeenth and eighteenth centuries that attitudes began to change and once more, the idea of bathing emerged from the shadows into which it had been banished. Gradually there emerged new fashions for both drinking and for bathing in the healing waters. Numerous health theories emerged which focused on cold water cures and the marvellous properties of heeling mineral spas. Books by Dr Floyer and Dr Oliver are examples of the more serious tomes of the 1700s, and John Wesley wrote his *Primitive Physick* which ran to twenty-one editions and was aimed at a less well-read audience.

It is worth differentiating here too, between bathing and swimming. The latter took place, if at all, in lakes, ponds and rivers and generally as a summertime leisure activity. However, for much of history, it is worth remembering that in a country such as England, very few people were swimmers. Water, and especially deep, cold water with undercurrents, was a potentially lethal hazard. The consequences of this risk and the increasing interest in summer swimming are noted in the annual Bills of Mortality. Here there are 104 'melancholy accidents' (i.e. drownings) recorded for one year in the 1700s. By the mid-1700s there were purpose-built swimming pools available in London: the Bagnio in Lemon Street, and the Peerless Pool in Finsbury. The latter offered both hot and cold baths and was developed from a natural pool popular with swimmers in the 1600s, but regarded then as a dangerous place to bath or swim. As it grew, the new facility offered swimming lessons, model boating, fishing, and in winter, ice skating. Like the Roman baths of old, there were other recreational and leisure activities on offer including reading rooms and exercise areas.

Bathing or swimming in the sea did not become popular until later. It took place in natural coastal pools and what were termed 'bathing holes' around the coast, but was not generally undertaken until after about 1750. Again, even fishermen were often unable to swim, and immersion in the sea frequently led to death by drowning.

With the Romans, it is apparent that bathing culture reached a peak that was not to be equalled or surpassed for over a thousand years after the fall of the Empire. The association between Roman civilisation and bathing is very strong. Despite their relative wealth and luxury, life was still short for most Romans; an expectancy of thirty years or so was about average. Furthermore, with very limited understanding of disease or illness and medicine, death could be quick and unexpected. Seemingly healthy individuals could become ill and die with frightening swiftness. Then, as was the case in early Western industrial societies in the 1700s and 1800s, medical treatises appeared which advocated healthy regimes and lifestyles to cure or avoid illness. Baths and bathing became central pillars of this pseudo-medicine and the role of these within the wider development of Roman medicine is far too great a subject to cover here. However, it is important to note the significance to the Romans of the association between bathing and good health. It is also worth considering that there is a difference between whether the Romans believed that their baths gave them good health, and indeed whether or not they really did so. Romans clearly felt that baths and bathing were good for them, but as I explain later, there were significant health risks too, and these were especially associated with poor water quality and lack of basic hygiene. A major opportunity for rebuilding in Rome, and for a new era of palatial bathhouses, arose around about AD 64, when, on 16 July during a moonlit night, the city burned. Just as was to happen in London in 1666, fire broke out in some shops on the Palatine and, fanned by a strong wind, spread to devastating effect across the city. Nero, far from the stuff of later myth, hurried back from nearby Antium to direct the fire-fighting and to oversee the provision of shelter for the newly homeless. The city of Rome was largely burned to the ground, but, like London in the 1600s, this provided a colossal opportunity for new building, and in this case it included major public baths. The new city was to be organised in a grid-like pattern of straight lines with a focus on the Emperor's magnificent palace – the 'Golden House', designed by the Imperial architects Severus and Celer. This luxurious design included pavilions, 100 hectares of parkland, temples, fountains, gardens, porticoes, and of course baths.

The major second-century medical writer Galen wrote abundantly on the health benefits of bathing. There are references to how baths and bathing might be used for curative purposes depending on particular circumstances. Earlier authors such as Pliny the Elder, Cornelius Celsus, Scribonius Largus, and others were already advocating bathing or medicinal purposes well before this time. Celsus, writing during the reign of Tiberius, gives a range of ailments for which a bathing regime might be increased or decreased as appropriate. These include fevers, liver problems, intestinal inflammation, small pustules, eye complaints, and both urinary and bowel problems. Communal bathing in untreated waters would consequently present huge issues of potential cross-infection and the spread of disease. Emperor Hadrian took steps to address this, and whilst he recognised the health benefits of bathing, reserved certain hours at the public baths in Rome for the exclusive use of the sick.

There are also many references by popular non-medical writers who advocated the health benefits of baths. Charmis of Massila apparently became very influential in Rome. As a promoter of the health-giving properties of cold-water baths, his writings led to even old men 'frozen stiff' as they stuck to his hydropathy guidance even in the depths of winter. At the other extreme, Pliny the Elder noted how Greek doctors had persuaded Romans to take boiling baths or *balinae ardentes* even when healthy. Indeed, the idea of baths and bathing being health-giving led to many incorporating regular baths into their daily routine even when in good health. A later author, Palladius, included comments on how bathing 'confers both great enjoyment and health'. The early Christian Church had to try and balance the obvious hedonistic pleasures of the baths, and their popularity, with its moral codes. The line it took was that baths were acceptable to visit but on hygiene and medical grounds rather than leisure and pleasure. Indeed, the bather should not enjoy the experience too much.

However, whatever the real benefits, baths and bathing became central to the perceived healthy lifestyle of educated Romans. If a man had become fatigued for some reason, then to maintain his health he should rest, and then take a bath. Other treatments were to sit by a warm fire or to sunbathe. Over time, the idea of therapeutic bathing came to sit alongside the bathhouse as a place of leisure and recreation in the Roman psyche. Bathing might be in water hot or cold, piped in or *in situ* at a spring or spa. However, there were and still are other ways of 'bathing' such as in mud or peat, or even in hot sand. The mud bath tradition goes far back into history. It is claimed that Cleopatra used Dead Sea black mud, and mud-therapies are found around the world. Wherever hot springs and volcanic ash appear together, there is the possibility of hot spring water but also hot mud. While the exact year of its inception is unknown, mud baths date back to the dawn of time. The ancient Romans incorporated the mud spa treatments into their bathing culture. It was both a preventative and a curative measure, and, as with bathing generally, it was also a socializing tool. The Roman villas where the hot muds naturally emanated were popular meeting places where members of the local community, men and women, old and young, healthy and sick, congregated to share lively conversation and above all, to immerse themselves in the health-giving mud.

The same draw of the medicinal muds and hot waters can be seen around the world today, from Eastern Europe to the United States of America. The mud baths grew in popularity in the United States in the 1940s and 1950s, as these ancient treatments enjoyed a revival. For obvious reasons the attraction was mostly with the elderly, seeking relief from arthritic and rheumatic suffering. A further growth in enjoyment of the mineral spas began in the 1970s, and continues to the present time. In Eastern Europe too, mineral springs and mud spas are hugely important and an accepted part of general care for health and well-being. These treatments have always crossed the lines between conventional medicine and ideas of natural healing. Above all, as it was for the Romans, the treatment is seen as the ultimate stress-reliever. Today in California for example, there is Calistoga, known as the 'mud bath capital' of North America. The mud is derived from volcanic activity linked to a major eruption of nearby Mount Konocti around eight million years ago which blanketed the area with rich, volcanic ash. The eruption resulted in cracks or fissures in the Earth's crust which mean that hot geysers and springs well up. The famous one is the Old Faithful Geyser, which is one of only three regularly erupting geysers in the world today. Here, as in the past, people gather to seek the healing waters and minerals.

In England, without any natural hot mud springs, the interest in bathing was largely focused on water and waters. Some spas have specialised in hot peat baths and bathing in imported muds, but the emphasis was on the spring waters. The English landscape is littered with spa place-names, and most of these derive from the heyday of the British spas in the 1700s and 1800s. However, there was also a long history of baths and watering-places which pre-dates this. Numerous spas enjoyed a reputation for healing waters and as water-places back into medieval times and in some case to the Romano-British and beyond. Certainly, throughout the medieval period many springs and wells were associated with healing properties and often with religious significance. Wells might be associated with a particular saint and visitors would sometimes have or at least claim to have had, visions of the Virgin Mary, and the like. However, in many cases these were springs and wells with ancient pagan associations and the Christian Church was simply trying to adopt them under its broad umbrella. It did a very similar thing with Christmas and that proved a great success!

Many wells or springs were dedicated to St Brigid which was a direct consequence of their former association with the Celtic goddess Brigantia. Why Brigantia, as a deity associated with arts and crafts, should have such ties with water and wells remains a mystery. In medieval England there were abundant well sites dedicated as shrines to Christian saints, but mostly with pagan origins. These were particularly common along the Celtic fringes of Cornwall and Wales, and in the northern regions of Northumbria and Cumbria. Individual sites and shrines were often dedicated to a saint and associated with miraculous events or visions. The more amazing or strong the event or miracle, then the more powerful would be the curative properties of the waters. Of course from the viewpoint of local people, the more amazing the visions and the stronger the cures, then the more opportunities there would be for financial benefit from visitors to the wells; an early form of religious tourism.

Also from early pagan times, wells had been decorated with flowers and garlands at local thanksgiving festivals. These were for the wells and the springs that spawned them and reflect the fact that water and the springs were at the centre of a local community and the lifeblood of its existence. In Derbyshire some of these well-dressings survive albeit under a Christian gloss. There are even places today which have well-dressings but certainly never had a well or at least not within any sort of memory; but they again, even if imaginary, become a great tourism draw. Droitwich, a Romano-British watering site, was famous as a centre of the salt trade and had a well dedicated to Saint Richard who was Richard de la Wyche, who apparently restored the important salt springs of the town. For many years the well was honoured and decorated to prevent it drying up in the future. Reputedly, when the well-dressing was abandoned at the order of the Parliamentarians during the Commonwealth, it did indeed dry up.

The fashionable healing spa at Gilsland in Cumbria was famed for its healing waters; so much so that a local entrepreneur bought the site and the surrounding land and built a house over the head of the well. However, the waters immediately dried up until the house was demolished, when they apparently ran again. This could be attributed to a spiritual upset or perhaps even a rational hydrological explanation. However, the later development of the spa facilities apparently didn't offend the gods and the waters continued to run freely.

In medieval times some wells were dedicated and famed for the cure of a particular illness or ailment. In many cases the problem was eyesight, which with the limits of medicine at the time and the generally very poor standards of hygiene is something to be expected. The small northern town of Rotherham had an 'eye well', as did Malvern, Ludlow (a 'bubbling well'), and Bradford (the 'Holy Well'). For some reason Herefordshire was especially endowed with eye cures. Some wells claimed to cure almost any illness and these were often associated with spectacularly inexplicable miracles. For example, St Catherine's Well at Newark in Nottinghamshire was the scene of a terrible murder. The victim was Sir Everard Bevercote and he was killed in an outburst of anger by his companion Sir Guy Saucimer. The latter regretted his actions but as a consequence of his deed became leprous. Then, when bathing in the well, the leprosy was cured, and in thanks for his recovery he built a chapel to enclose the healing well. The all-healing powers of the waters attracted pilgrims from far and wide. Many of the religious associations, some medieval and others pre-Roman Druidic legends, were suppressed or lost after the Reformation and the suppression of the Catholic Church with its emphasis on shrines. However, some healing waters continued in use from ancient times up to the present day.

2

ROMAN BATHS, SPAS, AQUEDUCTS & ENGINEERING

INTRODUCTION

Central to the possibility of bathing in a bathhouse was the ability to construct the necessary infrastructure to house and heat the water and to bring the water supply to the site, be it a city, a villa or a fort. This superior technology was at the core of Roman civilisation. The bath and the bathhouse were amongst the most obvious trappings of Roman luxury and civilisation. Evidence for the engineering, the construction and the management of these bathing facilities comes from written sources of the time, and also from the archaeology and monuments or artefacts where they survive. As the Roman Empire flourished and spread, and new ideas, designs and technologies became available, the bath grew from very modest origins to become a major focus of social and military lives. The bathhouses developed from rather minor features and into some of the most important examples of public architecture in Roman civilisation. Generally, the baths constructed in the more remote parts of the Empire, such as for example, in Britain, would be more modest than those of the great Roman metropolis. Even so, as the archaeology confirms, they could be important and significant buildings.

HEATING THE ROOMS AND THE WATER

A heated room would be a logical addition to the facilities in order to encourage perspiration and cleansing. Warmth was provided by external heating like an oven, a fire inside the room that might be raked out after pre-heating, or a charcoal brazier burning within the chamber. These hot, dry sweat rooms were named *laconia* after the Spartans of Laconia. The bathhouse heating was provided through the floors, the walls and even, in some cases, the ceiling vaults. The thermal baths at Aquae Sulis are one of the best known examples of heating through vaults and semi-domes in the ceiling. The system evolved to give clear separation between hot and cold rooms, and the various other functions of the bathhouse spaces. Sophisticated Roman technology allowed fine gradations of controlled conditions between rooms depending on their functions.

The key innovation of the Roman bathhouse was in the under-floor heating which warmed the very tiles on which the bathers walked. The word hypocaust means 'fire underneath' and refers to the use of a suspended floor, beneath which, and between the supporting pillars, could pass hot air and gases from a fire. The most basic structure was essentially a series of crude canals through which hot air passed. Variants on this system can be traced in Mediterranean cultures to perhaps 300 or 400 BC. The idea probably began with the Greeks but was developed to perfection by the Romans. The name is of Roman origin around about the first century AD, and the structures were somewhat like pottery kilns. Hot air and other gases emanated from an external fire or furnace stoked with fuel from outside, passed under the floor and then through the room itself, to exit via a hole in the roof. The conduits sloped upwards away from the furnace to help draw the hot air and gases into the main spaces. A bronze disc suspended below the exit hole in the roof could control the temperature of the room. By means of chains from which the disc hung, it could be raised or lowered to increase or decrease the temperature as required. Smaller, shallow trays were used as braziers to burn charcoal (a clean heat source) to control temperatures in particular spaces and smaller rooms. Fortunately, for the Roman bathers, the furnaces and braziers employed were designed to burn very efficiently and to produce carbon dioxide on combustion rather than the extremely poisonous and potentially lethal carbon monoxide. The hot room floors could be too hot to walk on in comfort, which suggests a temperature of around 42–44°C, to give an ambient room temperature of about 37–38°C. This is about right to produce the desired sweat.

As bath design evolved, clay pipes were used to act as chimneys and so to vent the hypocaust gases to the outside rather than through the room itself. The chimney design would also ensure a draught sufficient to draw the air over the fire and aid combustion. Examples of these sorts of features are found in the Roman remains in cities such as Pompeii and Herculaneum. By the last century BC, the Romans had evolved relatively complex bathhouses with what we would today regard as a 'Turkish Bath' provision. With a suite of rooms, these were presented as a gradation of temperature and humidity from an unheated room, to a warm room, and finally a hot steamy chamber. The baths were suspended on supporting pillars or hypocausts below, which, as described earlier, allowed the hot air to circulate. Cassius Dio suggested that the first public *laconicum* in Rome was built for Agrippa in 33 BC and the first heated swimming pool by Maecenas in 8 BC.

Of course, the Roman bathhouse designers had only limited understanding of either engineering or science. Concepts of things like humidity or precise quantitative measures of say temperature would have eluded them. In all probability, they simply produced the hypocaust structures and experimented until they worked effectively. Examination of the remains of bathhouses indicates that they experimented and added extra furnaces or enlarged existing ones, and added flues or other features until the desired effects were achieved. However, despite the limited understanding of any scientific principles, the Romans were able to arrive at quite sophisticated solutions to difficult problems, for example condensation. Anyone with a bathroom will understand the difficulties of controlling unwanted moisture and the associated damage it causes. Yet by the latter part of the first century BC, Roman designers had developed a form of dry-lining with tiles called *tegulae mammatae* or 'tiles with nipples'. With four perforated, conical lugs on one side, each close to a tile corner, when fastened to the wall surface, they provided a cavity. Nails hammered through the lugs and into the wall behind attached them, and the whole surface was then plastered over. It was possible to fix tiles so easily in this way because in much of Italy the building walls were made of volcanic tufa, similar in strength and texture to modern-day breeze blocks. Nails are easily driven into such a material.

This helped prevent both rising damp and condensation. Having mastered the idea of a cavity behind the walls to combat damp, the next step was to connect this same space with that below the flooring and to facilitate the flow of hot air and other gases up and around the room. The result would be the effective all round heating of the chamber. Furthermore, the walls with this modification became the main agents for heating the room, and because the tiles were relatively thin, the heat was transferred to the chamber more effectively.

When styles of buildings and the use of materials changed this presented problems for the designers. A move to concrete walls faced by tiles caused particular difficulties. The solution was a simple earthenware pipe called a *tubulus*. Archaeologists describe these as 'box-flue tiles' and they can stand against a wall without being physically fixed to it. The next step, maybe around the first century AD, was to key the tile face by combing or impressing a pattern into the surface before firing. Once this was achieved then the tiles could be fixed to the wall with mortar and plasterwork applied over the top.

There was even an unexpected benefit of this new system of heating, and this was associated with the sensitivity of the human body to radiant heat. This acts separately from the effects of the ambient air temperature around us. Imagine for example how quickly we feel warm with, say, an electric fire even before it has significantly raised the air temperature. The opposite but equally tangible effect is felt when the sun disappears behind a cloud on a hot summer's day. The air temperature is constant but you immediately feel cooler. The same effect happened as the wall tiles radiated heat into the chamber of the room. This meant that you got the same heating effect but at a lower room temperature. Once the Romans had realised the possibilities then they experimented with various different designs to produce the varied effects that were required.

STYLE AND FASHION

With the various changes in style and design, and particularly with the efficiencies of the wall-tile hypocausts, the baths could be operated at lower and more comfortable temperatures. They could be made bigger and even began to incorporate larger windows. Roman writer Seneca described a bath in a luxurious villa around AD 63 formerly owned by a man called Scipio:

> The bath is narrow and dark in the old-fashioned manner, for our forefathers equated heat with obscurity ... In this tiny corner he bathed a body weary with work in the field. But who nowadays could bear to bathe in this fashion? ... In this bath of Scipio's there are tiny slits – you can scarcely call them windows – cut through the stone wall so as to let in the light without weakening the fortifications. Nowadays, however, people regard baths as being only fit for moths if they have not been arranged so that they admit the sun through the widest of windows all day, and if men cannot get a sun tan and bathe at the same time, and look out from their tubs over the land and the sea.

This gives a vivid insight into how baths had been in the recent past but also how they were now perceived. It is also important to remember that whilst the Romans did have glass, it was not translucent and you would certainly not get a suntan through it, and neither would you have a clear view to the outside.

Seneca's description goes on: 'We know that certain devices have come to light in our own times, such as ... suspended baths with pipes set into their walls for the purpose of diffusing the heat and maintaining an even temperature from top to bottom ... All these kinds of things have been invented by the lowest slaves.' This last comment is a reminder that the whole social and economic system of the Roman Empire, like all other societies at the time, depended largely on slaves and slave labour.

As technologies progressed during the first century AD, the old narrow dark baths became obsolete. Increased efficiency due to the heated walls and other modifications to the hypocaust meant it was possible to warm much larger spaces, and with radiant heat, the ambient temperatures could be lower. At the same time, it was possible and became fashionable to include large windows, preferably with good views to the outside. For the Romans in their native Mediterranean haunts, this was all possible and the bathhouses became in part a sun lounge, heated by hypocausts, open to one side and heated by the sun. In the more northerly climes of the Empire, this was more challenging. It seems that in the colder regions it was the practice, if there were large windows, for them to be glazed. In order to conserve heat when necessary, it is likely that many of these windows were also shuttered.

PLANNING AND DESIGN

Clearly, the great public baths, the *thermae*, developed organised designs and conventions. In the provinces however, and amongst domestic baths, there was more innovation and variation. Many baths, especially in the Roman provinces, were built according to individual taste or need rather than to any accepted conventions. This is despite the standardisation of the basic units within a bath suite and the centralised manufacture of many of the component parts. The exceptions to this individuality are the bathhouses of great towns or of the Roman garrison forts for which there is a degree of similarity and standardisation.

All bathhouses, be they in a large villa or in a military fort would have the same basic principal chambers: a cold room or *frigidarium*, a warm room or *tepidarium*, and a hot room or *calidarium*.

THE COLD ROOM OR *FRIGIDARIUM*

This chamber was unheated and in some bathhouses probably served as a changing room, in others there was a separate changing room or *apodyterium*. However, the main function of the cold room was to be a place in which the bather could cool down after the hot rooms. This is necessary since following a very hot bath or time in a hot steam room for example, the human body experiences physiological inertia. Furthermore, dilation of the surface capillaries of the bloodstream causes lowered blood pressure, ruddy or flushed skin colouration, and deprivation of blood supply to vital organs. This effect, along with perspiration, may continue for some time after bathing and/or exercise. Therefore the cold room was designed to be a place in which the bather could cool slowly, or perhaps take a cold bath or a cold shower. The room generally would have a cold bath – *baptisterium*, or *puteus* – provided. Although such baths were often referred to as 'plunge baths', many were far too small to actually 'plunge'. These cold baths were typically about 0.7 metres deep and 1.0 metre across. It seems that the bather might have water poured over him or her whilst either standing or sitting on a step. Some baths – *piscina*, *natatio*, or *natatorium* – were larger and facilitated full immersion or even swimming.

THE WARM ROOM OR *TEPIDARIUM*

In the warm room the bather could begin to prepare and acclimatise for the really hot conditions of the hot room. It is likely that the temperature was at or about 40°C, which is slightly above ambient body temperature, and physiological inertia is overcome to produce the onset of perspiration and vascular or capillary dilation. A servant or slave would anoint the bather with cleansing oils. In some cases the oils were applied in a special room called the *unctorium* or *the elaeothesium*, literally the place for the application of unguents.

THE HOT ROOM OR *CALIDARIUM*

The central part of the bathing experience would be the hot room or *calidarium*, in which the temperature was maintained high, perhaps at about 60°C like a modern Turkish bath. The tiled floor of such a room would be far too hot to touch unprotected. Wooden-soled sandals or *soleae balneares* were worn to protect the feet from the heat. Injury through burning on the hot surfaces of floors or walls was not unknown, and apparently when his slaves tried to kill him, Larcius Macedo's slaves threw him onto the hot floor to see if he was just pretending to be dead.

The hot room was also humid and for smaller baths a separate concrete hot tank (or steam tank) was provided over the furnace to supply the steam. The bather in the hot room could wash his or her face with either warm water or cold water from a basin or *labrum* on a pedestal. This was often located within a semi-circular apse or *schola*.

Once the bather was cleansed by scraping off the oils with a strigil then they would bathe in a hot bath known as an *alveus*, *piscina calida* or *solium*. Some of the baths were maintained at very high temperatures. Senecca described the hot baths as 'being on fire', and suggested, tongue-in-cheek, that a slave convicted of a criminal act should be bathed alive as punishment. On leaving the hot room the bather returned to the cold room to cool down in comfort.

THE SWEAT CHAMBER OR *LACONICUM*

Some bathhouses included a further hot room, in which the temperature was even higher than the ordinary hot room. Here the room was hot and dry, and named *laconicum* after Laconica, the homeland of the Spartans. These rooms are sometimes called a *sudatorium* (meaning 'I sweat'), but that can be applied to both humid and dry rooms.

OUTSIDE THE BATHS

A bathhouse complex might include exercise areas or yards similar to early gymnasia or palaestra. These were somewhat similar to a cloister, a colonnaded courtyard. A covered *basilica* or hall housed further facilities for leisure and relaxation.

THE FURNACE ROOM

A vital part of the provision of the bathhouse experience was the means of providing heat, the furnace. This was an arched tunnel that went underneath the wall from the outside of a heated room. The stokers generally were in a separate and unconnected space from the baths, in their own room called a *praefurnium*. It is believed that the fire burned almost like a simple bonfire, without any grate and seated simply on the floor of the tunnel. Whilst this lack of technological sophistication seems surprising, a fire made like this will burn for a long time even when unattended. It is also easy to rake out the ashes. This seems to have been the standard approach used even in industrial furnaces. The temperature of the burn is also easily controlled by straightforward adjustments to the size and shape of the fire. Burning the fire causes air to be drawn into the tunnel and so into the hypocaust, the rate of inflow depending on the difference in temperature between the air outside and the hot gases at the bottom of the wall flues. As the temperature below the floor gets higher, more air is drawn over the furnace fire and the rate of heating drops. This is a different effect from that which would happen if the fire burned in a grate. If more air was pulled through, then the fire would burn more strongly and, a positive feedback loop, the temperature would rise further. However, it is possible to raise the temperature in a simple fire by means of bellows which force the air through the fuel rather than allowing it to pass over the top. Some of the furnaces for bathhouses have other channels and drain-like structures but it is not known what these might have done.

FUEL

Generally it appears that the Romans used wood to heat their hypocausts. Mineral coal, available from surface outcrops and coastal sites, was burnt in some parts of Britain and is found associated with hypocausts, but not specifically with baths. A major problem with burning mineral coal, although this varies between outcrops, is the amount of impurities. This would be a distinct disadvantage to any burning which might release gases into a room-space. Of particular concern would be incomplete combustion and the potential for the release of lethal carbon monoxide. Wood charcoal may also have been used and indeed has many advantages of cleanliness and uniformity of temperature when compared with other fuels. Since charcoal also has a higher rate of energy release per unit weight, it requires less storage space. The key thing with charcoal is that it produces very little smoke – a distinct advantage in a system where fumes may permeate into the bathing rooms.

Without precise information on the usage and the methods employed it is impossible to calculate exactly how much fuel a particular bathhouse might have consumed. However, if the furnace burnt wood, it was mostly supplied by managed coppice, a system that is attributed to the Romans. Coppice wood is cut on a regular fifteen- to twenty-five-year cycle and the regrown stems are harvested, cut and dried for burning. This may be as wood or as charcoal. It is likely that a significant part of a Roman agricultural estate might be set to producing coppice wood fuel. A calculation for the small bathhouse at Welwyn in Hertfordshire is quoted by Tony Rook (2002). With rooms 2.4 metres square it is suggested that the site would have used the coppice wood produced from around 23 hectares of managed woodland.

The costs of keeping the baths fuelled could be very high and this was something that a benefactor might sponsor. The writer Miletus put it rather nicely, that the baths operated when 'the fire-wedded nymphs' were summoned. A wealthy benefactor might establish a foundation to pay for the wood used for heating, or even agree that coppice woodland on his estate be harvested to supply the fuel. At Misenum there was an arrangement for 400 wagon-loads of wood to be given to heat the baths each year. This was further passed to the town's magistrates to ensure that the practice continued into the future to be overseen by their successors. Repairs to worn-out infrastructure also gave opportunities for generous bequests to in part elevate the donor's public status. In some cases too, the local council administered moneys to purchase private bathhouses and make them public.

CONSTRUCTING THE BUILDINGS

Another major innovation in Roman building, which also had a big impact on bathhouses, was the invention of concrete. One of the key developments in architecture was to use vaults and arches, employed by the Ancient Egyptians and the Greeks, but only for underground structures. Previously all aboveground buildings relied on post and lintel, or column and architrave constructions with straight lines. Roman design changed all this and it brought curves from underground to be visible features in their architecture. The other change from say Greek construction, was that instead of planning the stone blocks to be a perfect fit, the Romans cut blocks more roughly and fitted them together using mortar. The latter was effectively an artificial mud made from sand and slaked lime mixed together with water.

In creating their curved arches, the Romans employed a series of cut, tapered stone blocks which when fitted together, formed the arc of a circle. This allowed wider expanses to be bridged when a solid stone block, as well as being heavy and unwieldy, would also be prone to fracture. Stone has limited strength in tension and so a single beam may be vulnerable to catastrophic failure. However, stone is instead very strong under compression, and so the cut blocks of the arch, or *voussoirs,* provide strong support. Their natural tendency is to splay the structure outwards and so, in order to keep the building intact, strong buttresses are provided to support the arch. The stone blocks were generally finished with mortar. Because sand was not so easily available over much of Roman Italy, the slaked lime was often mixed with powdered volcanic ash to produce something very similar to Portland cement. This powdered ash was called *pozzolana*, after Pozzuoli just north of Naples where the material was quarried. When ash was unavailable, the Romans improvised with powdered tiles.

Unlike other great public buildings, which had accepted and established forms, the bathhouses could be subject to considerable architectural innovations. Many of the new designs and ideas developed in the great public bathhouses. In the great Roman metropolis, with grand baths built by emperors and with free admission, the buildings became publicly accessible palaces with leisure and recreation available on a regal scale. As such, the great public baths grew to be the focus of social and cultural life in the city. Nero had *thermae,* or hot baths, constructed at Campus Martius. Others were built or started by Trajan, Titus, Antonius, Diocletian, and Constantine.

THE HYPOCAUST

The first usage of the term hypocaust was by Vitruvius in the first century AD, even though such systems and structures were used well before then, by both Romans and Greeks. In its earliest use it is most closely translated as a 'furnace': 'Three bronze boilers are to be set over the hypocaust, one for hot, one for tepid, and one for cold water ... The arrangement must allow the heat exchangers for the bath tubs to be heated by the same hypocaust.' In the later first century, a poem by Statius describes the heating of the room from below: 'languidly creeps the warmth about the house, while a faint haze rolls up from the hypocaust beneath.' This gives a nice feel of the luxury and comfort of Roman living.

The stokehole and other spaces beneath the heated rooms were generally excavated to a depth of about one metre. Sometimes they were floored with tiles or flagstones, but often they were just earth floors. In order to support the floors of the heated rooms above, there were short columns or *pilae* spanning the 1-metre gap. These columns were often made from square 20-centimetre-wide tiles stacked on top of each other. Placed on the columns was a floor of flags, each about 0.6 metres diameter, and then a final surface of tiles or mosaic was added.

CHIMNEYS

As noted earlier, the original bathhouses simply vented via a hole in the roof. However, for reasons of practicality and of comfort, the system soon evolved to include venting of gases and hot air to the outside via a chimney. As hot air and gases passed through the hypocaust and up the insides of the walls, they escaped to the outside through vents or chimneys. From around AD 100 onwards, the most common form of flue was a structure called a *tubulus* used either across the whole of the wall or in a set of vertical slots. The vent to the exterior was probably set high in the building and perhaps just under the eaves of the roof. It is likely that there was a lot of variation and the builder probably experimented until a suitable and workable system was in place. Some domestic bathhouses, as discovered at Pompeii, had vertical chimney pipes.

Despite the efforts of the builder, it is likely that Roman bathhouses did suffer from noxious fumes emanating from the boiler house and the associated pipework. Gases and smells from the furnaces could and did get to the bathing rooms and could inconvenience bathers. Indeed, it was even the case that in some instances where a bathhouse manager wished to clear out undesirables, they threw darnel grass seed onto the hot coals. This produces a gas which caused dizziness and headaches and so encouraged the unwanted clientèle to leave. Other writers complain about smoke and fumes in the bathhouses heated by furnaces. Some of the comments are made specifically about what were quite up-market establishments, so it is likely that the lower end of the market was much worse. It is suggested that in large public bathhouses with large amounts of fuel being burnt to heat the buildings and the waters, smoke and fumes would be commonplace. This would not be manifested as rooms filled with smoke, but more as insidious background seepage of smell and gas through walls, floors, and conduits into the public spaces.

CAPPING IT OFF – CEILINGS AND ROOFS

The innovation of vaulted rooms and arches has already been discussed, and it was normal for bathhouse to have bathrooms with vaulted ceilings. In order to make this possible for larger buildings, the Roman engineers utilised lightweight materials to construct the vaults. Hollow *voussoirs* or trapezoid *tubuli* were employed along with *voussoirs* of calcareous tufa, and hollow ribs of tiles or tufa. It is possible that these hollow, light-weight structures might have had a double function and allowed further circulation of the hot gases.

BRINGING WATER TO THE BATH

Early Roman bathhouses and facilities not served by aqueducts relied on modest local sources of water-supply. This would involve both obtaining water and some means of storing it until use. Often there would be a simple pipeline from a nearby spring or other water source, but some baths relied on water from a well collected in buckets. Some later baths had large water-wheels to lift considerable volumes of water to storage reservoirs for subsequent use. Wheels up to 7 metres in diameter were known.

Some baths in the cities were supplied direct from great storage cisterns which housed the township's water-supply; others required their own aqueducts. The latter were generally the most reliable and effective way to supply water to a large public bathhouse. In order to maintain the great imperial *thermae*, a continuous and substantial supply of water was required. This meant thousands of litres of water provided by extensive aqueducts and is one of the great engineering feats of Roman civilisation. At one point the City of Rome received a million gallons of water per day via nine major aqueducts; a supply equivalent to around 300 gallons per person per day. On the other hand, a small villa bathhouse might be kept supplied by slaves with buckets. Once on site, water could be moved by means of pumps such as an Archimedes screw, a drum or cylinder pump, or a bucket and chain.

The remains of aqueducts and other structures bear testimony to the sophistication of this engineering. For example, the Roman city of Lindum Colonia or Lincoln has, just inside the city wall, a Roman Reservoir. It is suggested that whilst people dug wells and collected rainwater for everyday needs, this could not supply all the necessary communal works such as the public bathhouse. To solve the problem therefore, a pipeline was constructed, extending north eastwards for over a kilometre, to a spring known as Roaring Meg. The pipe itself was made of clay and encased in *opus signinum*, powdered tile mortar. A bridge was built to carry the aqueduct though there are problems of levels and it is likely that pumping was also required. Smaller pipes were made of earthenware pottery, wood sections joined by iron collars, or lead.

Hot water would be supplied to the baths by boilers placed over the furnaces. These were usually made of bronze or lead with copper bottoms, and then encased in concrete. Looking somewhat like milestones they were actually called *millaria* because of this. Basic plumbing was constructed from lead and taps were made of cast bronze. A long-term consequence of their extensive water-supplies, provided down lead pipes, may have been lead poisoning of the Roman people. By means of branched pipes and paired taps, hot and cold water could be mixed to the required temperature. This task would be undertaken by the attendant working at the stoke-hole. Large iron beams found at some sites may have been used to support the weight of the boiler.

DRAINAGE

With so much water and the number of visitors, the bathhouses would require drains. In some cases, these were simple ditches, but in other locations, they were lined gullies or even pipes. Waste water from the baths was used to flush out the latrines. When a facility included latrines, they were a series of perforated seats placed over an open gully.

MAINTENANCE AND REPAIR

There was a world of difference between the modest neighbourhood bathhouse boasting a few warm and tidy rooms and the great Imperial *thermae* of the metropolis. The latter would offer the patron a diversity of rooms and spaces, indoors and out, for bathing, exercise, and other entertainments. The more modest *balneae* provided for a simple ritual of bathing and socialising, whereas the *thermae* gave enjoyment for the masses and often as a grand gesture, a gift from the Emperor. Whilst many bathhouses made a charge for their use, others were free. Baths were constructed in such great numbers across the empire because they were popular and the demand was huge. As the culture of bathing grew, then the construction and running of bathhouses became a good economic proposition. They made good money and there were obvious business opportunities on the side such as catering and more. The buildings or complexes of buildings might include lecture rooms, exercise halls, libraries, religious cult shrines, porticoes, promenades, gardens, palaestrae, and running tracks for athletes. This provision was alongside the hot and cold baths themselves. However, bathhouses were notoriously difficult and expensive to maintain and so running these 'people's palaces' was a costly business. The combinations of heat and water would wreak havoc with masonry, plasterwork, and the pipe and duct systems. Often they fell into disrepair, and this also provided opportunities for public-spirited, wealthy individuals to make donations for their repair. This might raise their public standing and it perhaps also placed them in a favourable light with the appropriate gods. Lead was vital to the functioning of the water systems and a benefactor at Nemus Dianae in Italy was noted as giving a quantity of lead to the 'old bath' for the repair and maintenance of the bathhouse.

The council at Lanuvium constructed a new suite of *thermae* to replace the old *balneae* because of their poor condition. The situation was described whereby 'through old age' they had ceased to be used. Similarly at Antium, the bathhouse decayed so severely that people were deterred from using them because they were hazardous. It is clear from the writings and dedications related to repairs and bequests for maintenance or rebuilding that a bathhouse that was once a splendid and fine building could degenerate quite quickly. These were buildings that were well used, had hot water and steam as essential features, and had elaborate designs and decorations unsuited to such extreme conditions. Again the writings of the time make it clear that many baths struggled to maintain the standards they had at the time of their opening. Inscriptions refer to the bathhouses being restored to their original appearance and note that for long periods the facilities had been in poor condition.

A big issue for the bathhouse concept is its relationship to health and hygiene. With limited understanding of disease or disinfection, and limited technologies in terms of supplying and purifying water, the bathhouses, far from being places to generate health, could be death-traps. Even the grand buildings might be far short of our modern concepts and expectations of hygiene and cleanliness. Water quality itself might be a real problem. Whilst Seneca noted that bathers in his time were fastidious about water purity, the reality might have been very different. Frontius for example, stated that the Roman baths of the Republican time were supplied by water from public troughs. After heavy rain the water was muddy and sometimes the supplies brought by various aqueducts were mixed by the water men, or *aquarii,* and as a result they all became cross-contaminated and sub-standard. This was a problem for both drinking water and for bathing. Some bathhouses note steps taken to find supplies from, say, a pure spring, but the implication is that for a long time previously, the water was impure.

Once the water arrived at the bathhouse, then communal bathing and immersion would further affect quality and hygiene. With only rudimentary knowledge of disease and illness, some health issues would become obvious. Celsus for example, noted that it was ill-advised to visit the bathhouse with a fresh wound or one that had not been properly cleaned. He suggests that in making the wound both wet and dirty, the result could be gangrene. Indeed, the hazards of communal bathing in the *solium* were described by Martial when he wrote: 'Zoilus, you spoil the *solium* by washing your arse. To make it filthier, Zoilus, stick your head in it.' He goes on: 'You don't like anyone to wash in the *solium* before yourself, Cotilus. What is the reason except that you would rather not be laved by irrumated water? But though you are first in the bath, it needs must be that your cock is washed here before your head.' Furthermore, he chastises another bather: 'You bathe as though you were angry with the public, Charidemus, washing your groin all over the *solium*. I wouldn't have you wash your head here like that, Charidemus. There now, you're washing your head. I'd sooner you washed your groin.' He gives a pithy impression of what conditions might have been like and the problems of washing in someone else's filth.

The combination of questionable water quality at the outset, and then the obvious issue of communal bathing and washing, make for a very unhygienic experience. Martial also describes how bathers would enter the communal pools caked in muds and oils from their treatment and preparation in the bathhouse. All this gunge would add to the general filth in the waters. Furthermore, with no chemical disinfectants in the waters, and sometime very irregular changing of the bathwater, in individual tubs or pools, the conditions could become quite bad. Many baths did have a constant supply of running water and this created an overflow onto the surrounding floor tiles. However, given time and a lack of disinfection, this system would also provide ample opportunities for microbes and other organisms to flourish. Additionally, the through-flow of water would not necessarily sweep foul water out to the deep pools. Bathhouses were regularly inspected by the authorities in an attempt to keep an eye on the owners and managers who might otherwise be tempted to cut corners in hygiene and cleanliness.

There have been suggestions as to the frequency of the changing of bathwater such as at the cistern-fed baths at Rhodiapolis (Farrington in Fagan, 1999). This was suggested to be once a week or twice every three weeks. Together with the absence of chemical treatments, this indicates that the bathhouse might not be particularly hygienic, and certainly not by comparison with today's standards. There are ways to minimise risks to health as employed in the Japanese hot pools for example. In this case, washing rather than bathing is undertaken separately, with buckets of water taken from the communal pool and poured over the bather. However, there is no evidence to suggest that the Romans did this, so we can safely assume that they washed and bathed together in these rather unclean communal baths. In modern public baths the processes of disinfection and of hygiene are seen as essential to the proper running of such a facility. This was not the case in Roman times.

The physical cleaning of the baths and bathhouses is also interesting since it was sometimes undertaken by convicted criminals used as public servants; perhaps something akin to modern-day 'community service' sentences. The bathhouse buildings would accumulate mess and filth from people and their activities. The cleansing process of 'strigiling', scraping oil from the body with a strigil must have caused a mix of sweat, dirt, oil and skin to be dripped or splashed onto floors and walls. The medical writer Aetius Amidenus collected the material from baths and water to use as a binding agent in his medicines. The ease with which he could do this suggests something in terms of the state of the buildings and the water. It was this condition that promoted the idea of bathhouse cleaning as a punishment. In particular, the job of cleaning the hypocaust with its metre-high spaces must have been especially gruelling.

In human habitations where there are people and activities, there is often the likelihood of vermin. The eminent Roman writer Pliny the Elder noted the bathhouses to be the breeding grounds of cockroaches.

It is probable that the Roman bathhouses spanned the broad range from grandly decorated and highly maintained splendour, to dirty, seedy and dilapidated. Buildings and provision which began life in splendour would, without adequate maintenance, descend into conditions far from those anticipated by their builders and their users. In comparison with the expectations of today, even the grandest baths would have presented conditions far below acceptable levels of sanitation. Whilst the Romans considered the baths important in terms of health, hygiene, and cleanliness, the modern reader must be aware that the thresholds of acceptability were much lower than we have today. Such ideas of hygiene and cleanliness are relative rather than absolute, and the Romans were relatively clean. Marcus Aurelius asked, 'What is bathing when you think about it – oil, sweat, filth, greasy water, everything loathsome.'

3

BATHS & BATHING IN ROMAN CULTURE

The bath and bathing were important to Romans in terms of cleanliness – and this separated them from the smelly barbarians, but they were much more than this. Not only central to urban sophisticated living, the baths were vital for the military too; as places for relaxation, cleaning and for exercise and training. A visit to Caerleon in South Wales brings home vividly the importance of these facilities to a Roman legion abroad. The Imperial *thermae* in Rome were magnificent structures with soaring, valued roof-spaces and ground-breaking architecture. The complexes spread across city blocks to include gardens and parks and other associated features and facilities. At the other end of the scale of lavishness would have been the simple rural *balneae* of a modest Romano-British villa, or the communal bathhouse of a legionary outpost.

The origins of bathing were entirely functional rather than leisurely. People bathed to get clean rather than to enjoy the experience. There were also significant differences in bathing practice from what we expect today. Soap for example, was not used by the Roman bathers, only being invented somewhat later by Germanic peoples. Pliny mentioned German soap in the first century AD, and even gives a recipe for making it: 'soap is also good; an invention of the Gallic provinces for making hair red, it is made from suet and ash in two kinds – the best from beech ash and goat suet …' The possible effect on hair colour seems to have discouraged its use by many Romans.

In order to cleanse the body, along with water both hot and cold, the Romans and Greeks used the application of oils, often with fuller's earth and pumice. The oil was applied to the body, often massaged in, and then removed by scraping off with a special curved instrument called a strigil.

The latter are known to have been in use from as early as the sixth century BC. To maximise the efficacy of the oil cleansing it was good to have the skin perspiring either due to exercise or through high temperature in the sweat-house. It is likely that the Greek gymnasium or palaestra, a wrestling school, had associated baths and the athletes cleansed with oils, strigils and then washed with water. At least some of these facilities included hot water. Greek baths were designed to sit in and have water poured over you, whereas the earlier baths of the Minoans and Mycenaeans were built to allow submersion. The Etruscans are also believed to have used sweat rooms.

In the times of the Republic, public bathing was generally considered to be morally unacceptable, but by AD 33 there were at least 170 public baths just in Rome itself. However, even so, men and women bathed separately. From remains at Pompeii, it seems that there were separate bathing suites for men and women. Later designs of larger bathhouses are often symmetrical and it may be that although not physically separated, men used one half and women the other. The shared axis of the design was usually a shared swimming pool. By this time, mixed bathing had become accepted practice until it was prohibited by a decree of the Emperor Hadrian during the second century AD. The rules on separate bathing were later restated by both Marcus Aurelius (in the latter part of the first century) and Severus Alexander (in the second century AD). This need for reaffirmation is taken to imply that the guidance was often ignored.

The first public baths in Rome were built as two buildings, one for men and one for women, but connected so as to share the heating furnace and ducts. Others such as at Pompeii and Herculaneum also had double facilities. As well as designing bathhouses for dual usage, the other solution to mixed use was for the two sexes to frequent them at different times. This was certainly the case with some public baths and the sexes each had shifts of maybe seven or eight hours. It is not always clear whether non-segregated establishments were indeed used for mixed bathing or there was a time-share arrangement. By the second century AD, it was commonplace to meet high-born ladies naked in the mixed baths. However, a prohibition on mixed bathing issued by Emperor Hadrian was perhaps a move to try and control the increasing number of sexual scandals in Roman society at the time. By the time of Emperor Alexander Severus (AD 225–35), there was even a *balnea feminarum* or ladies' bath, watched over by eunuchs. This almost presages the Ottoman Seraglios of a later era.

For the Romans, their baths were more than places for cleaning and washing. They had become the great focus for social and cultural activities.

The writer Seneca provides a feel for the social melee of the public bathhouse:

> I'm in the midst of a roaring babel. My lodgings are over the baths! Imagine every possible outcry to shatter your eardrums. When the more athletic bathers swing their dumbbells I can hear them grunt as they strain, or pretend to, and hissing and gasping as they expel their breath after holding it. There's a lazy chap happy with a cheap massage; I hear the smack of the hand on his shoulders, the sound varying with whether it strikes flat or cupped. If an umpire comes to keep score at the ball game, counting the tosses, it's all up with me!
>
> Now add the argumentative noisy pickpocket caught in the act and the sound of the man who loves to hear the sound of his own voice in the bath. After that, the people who jump in the pool with an almighty splash, besides those with raucous voices. You have to imagine the dipilator giving his falsetto shriek to advertise his presence and never silent except when making somebody else scream by plucking hair from his armpits. There's the refreshment man with his wide range of cries, the sausage vendor, the confectioner, the men from the places of refreshment shouting their wares, each with his own vendor's cry.

This wonderful description paints a vivid picture of the bathhouse scene that might be from modern times.

Alongside their functional construction, the imperial hot baths or *thermae* were decorated with works of art, mosaics, and exotic stones. They included exercise years, gardens and libraries. The grand urban designs also triggered the aspirations of wealthy Romans in the wider countryside. Therefore, the larger villas mimicked the grandeur of their urban public facilities to create '*urbs in rure*', the scale according to the means. This fashion extended from the rural Romans to the far reaches of the Empire; and in the provinces, the extent of bathhouse luxury was seen as a marker of Romanisation and civilisation.

The bathhouses were great social meeting places. Here, the great and the lowly might rub shoulders in a remarkably egalitarian breakdown of the otherwise class-ridden Roman society. Presumably there was some degree of segregation in terms of some people using the grand and lavish Imperial bathhouses and others tending to more modest provisions. Even the Emperors might visit and use the public baths, as testified by the story of Hadrian and the man rubbing his back against the wall (see later in this chapter). As well as visits from emperors, the bathhouses would include senators and other members of Rome's elite society. This is a dramatic example of social mixing in Roman society but one that was not always the case. Generally, it seems that an important person wanting to bathe would join in and mix in with the crowd; but this is not always the case. A notable exception was the case of a travelling consul whose wife wished to bathe and to do so privately but in the men's bathhouse at Teanum Sidicinum. Having ordered the baths to be cleared for her use, she had the local magistrate flogged for taking too long to comply with her demands. In response, a nearby town issued a decree to say that locals were to be banned from bathing if a Roman magistrate was in town. However, this example flouts the general trend and was taken as unpalatable upper-class arrogance. In most case, the baths were for the town's public and anybody could and did use them. If there was segregation of sorts, and this may well have been the situation, then it was most likely to be through access at different times of day. In Pompeii for example, it has been suggested that the baths were open only for the elite between the sixth and eighth hour. Others such as labourers or the owners of snack bars could use them later on. This does seem to be problematic since at the later hours, shopkeepers and snack bar owners would have been at their busiest. It would make more sense for them to bathe earlier in the day when business was quieter. Furthermore, there is an idea that the commoners only rarely used the hot baths. This was presumably because the hot baths cost more. Young aristocratic youths tended to wear an amulet or *bulla* as a mark of their social standing and freeborn nature. It has been suggested that this was to distinguish them from slaves and in part so that older men, happening on them naked in the baths, would not abuse or 'debauch' them as they might a slave.

For many common people of the larger Roman cities, living conditions were generally pretty squalid. With this in mind, the public bathhouses would be a relatively pleasant environment to visit and to hang around. Especially during cooler weather, these would be magnets to draw in the wider public. There was also the excitement of seeing the rich and famous and gaining some insight into how the others lived. Graffiti scribbling on bathhouse walls indicates the sorts of people who visited. In particular, it is clear that husbands and wives would visit the baths together, and also entire families including children would bathe, though perhaps not at every facility. Slaves were also present both as attendants to their masters and mistresses but also as bathers in their own right. In some cases a wealthy patron would attend with a number of slaves or servants carrying all sorts of paraphernalia for the bathing experience. Writers describe

Imperial and aristocratic visitors arriving at the baths with a retinue of fifty or more slaves and servants. It is probably unlikely that slaves were regular bathers at the public baths, but it is certainly the case that they could and did sometimes attend. The status of Roman slaves varied dramatically with owner and the position of the particular slave. In some cases to go outside the master's house without permission could incur a punishment of a hundred lashes. In other cases, slaves helped to run businesses and might be away from the main household for considerable periods. It is likely that these individuals would partake of the communal baths. Graffiti and other evidence can place a slave at the bathhouse but whether as a bather or merely an attendant is not always clear. There is an example of graffiti from Herculaneum that attests for a specific example of a slave partaking of the bathhouse experience. Apelles Mus, who describes himself as a 'chamberlain of the emperor' is noted as eating and enjoying sex at the baths along with his 'brother' Dexter. These were not brothers in blood but two senior imperial slaves partaking of what was Herculaneum's latest and most luxurious Suburban Baths. Overall it seems that slaves were able to use public baths as paying customers, but the practice varied from bath to bath, town to town and region to region.

Of course the bathhouses were not just patronised by residents, but would serve a wider populace from the countryside around. Farmers and other rural people would not attend the baths every day, but on market days, when there were festivals, local elections, or other special days, then they would descend on the town and use the facilities. They would no doubt look forwards with anticipation to, as an advertisement puts it, 'bathing in the manner of the city'. The relatively wealthy and sophisticated urbanites would then not only share their baths with the various social strata of the town, but with the influx of rustics wanting to taste the high life.

It is also unclear as to whether a patron of the baths paid extra to bring their slaves in attendance, or whether they were considered just part of the essentials of a visit like towels, strigils, and oils, etc. In some cases, baths were built in part for the specific use of slaves. When imperial baths were built for the use of locals and slaves serving the imperial estates in a particular region, this was certainly the case. There are other examples where it is clear that slaves and servants could and did use the baths and in some cases they bathed alongside those of higher social status. A Romano-British villa at Ashurst in Surrey was excavated and two baths were found; one a small bath for the family built into the main house and the other a larger structure some fifty metres down the approach road. The larger bath was for the estate workers. Not all British villas were so well provided for and in many cases the workers had to make do with the public facilities in the nearest village.

The Roman baths had many social functions and it has been argued that the intermingling and mixing of many people from the different social strata performed a role of social levelling. However, the bathhouse also provided a pace to flaunt one's wealth and status, arriving in pomp and ceremony and with a large entourage of attendants. Furthermore, the positioning of villas and houses in terms of proximity to the baths was also very important. Fine clothes and jewellery were worn throughout the experience of bathing, and in some cases patrons were borne around on litters, pampered with fine oils and unguents, and generally showed off their rank, status and wealth. The lower-ranking visitors would try to emulate their betters but often with little success. Whilst the idea of showing off appealed to some, others preferred a less public experience and the master might despatch his slave to survey the scene and check if the baths were not too busy, before he himself ventured out.

A wealthy bather would no doubt have slaves to clear the way before him as he progressed to the bathhouse. But even so, the prolixity to so many plebs and commoners was no doubt irritating and annoying. Slaves and servants would be employed to keep prying plebs away from the elite bathers, and here in the steamy pools, much business, politics and social networking would have been done. The bathhouse provided a place for mixing and to be seen, for socialising and for business, and for leisure and hygiene. However, whilst they facilitated interactions between the social strata in a confined space, they also reinforced the visible barriers and status between the levels of Roman society. The elite patrons would dine apart and on fine wine and better food. They were all members of the great Roman community, but the differentiation between the leaders and the led was visible and obvious. The bathhouse brought everyone together but it also played an important role in reinforcing social positions.

The bathhouses ranged from the great Imperial *thermae* to the abundant, small, urban baths of the city of Rome, with hundreds of baths from the exclusive and luxurious to the drab and dilapidated. The poets wrote in glowing terms about the wonderful and luxurious bathhouses but we should not forget that scattered throughout the poorer quarters there would be poorly designed and badly kept baths with few luxuries and little to recommend them. As noted later, many were served by especially poor-quality water and may have represented serious health hazards rather than places of therapy. Yet for the urban-dwelling Romans, the great bathhouses offered them chance to bathe in style and relative luxury. For many plebs, escaping from cramped housing and dusting streets, this may have been their only opportunity to bathe at all.

THE PROCESS OF BATHING

Pliny the Younger described very simply the actual steps in the bathing process: 'I am oiled, I take my exercise, I have my bath.' We also know of the routine for a schoolboy visiting the baths. He would arrive at the bathhouse with a slave or servant carrying the necessary bathing equipment and garments. Having paid the bath fee he would proceed to the changing rooms to undress and store his clothing. He would be oiled and anointed with perfumes and proceed to the sweat bath. This was followed by full immersion in the hot bath and then a swim in the cold bath which might be outside. His body would then be thoroughly dried by his attendant and then he would dress. Having bid farewell to others at the baths, he would thank the bath master and depart.

The wealthy patron arriving at the bathhouse would bring an entire retinue to bear him or her, plus the paraphernalia needed for bathing and for exercise. The bathing garments consisted of sandals and towels and there was also his or her *cista* or toilet kit. This was usually a cylindrical metal box containing oils and perfumes in flasks, a number of strigils to scrape oil from the body, and a sponge. The less affluent would carry their own garments and boxes, but since this was an exercise in public display, the wealthy would arrive with a large group of slaves and perhaps even be carried in a litter or sedan chair.

On arrival you undressed in the *apodyterium* or changing room. These probably had wooden boxes, chests, cabinets and benches for storage and for seating. Larger bathhouses would also be provided with shelves, niches and cubbyholes all built into the masonry structure. Some baths also had strong benches. Some of the smaller and lower-class establishments would just have wooden pegs on the wall for hanging your personal effects. Security was an issue and theft was not uncommon and is evidenced by curse tablets found at some baths to gain revenge on those responsible for thieving. The wealthier patrons simply posted a slave or servant to watch over their belongings whilst they bathed.

Generally, the bather would undertake some light exercise prior to the process of bathing. This was considered healthy and the guidance was to do just enough to raise a slight sweat. Public bathhouses would generally have facilities both indoors and out to undertake exercise. These were based on the Greek gymnasium, and were often colonnaded courtyards known as palaestrae. The patron intending to exercise before bathing would have changed into a light tunic designed for the purpose. Unlike the Greeks, the Romans did not exercise nude, and neither would they enter the hot rooms in their street clothing or shoes. Women might exercise in a skimpy garment somewhat like a bikini. There were also heavier cloth wraps to wear after exercise to protect you from the cold; probably essential in the more northerly parts of the Empire. Fashionable youths might also wear a tight-fitting cap to protect their hair from oil.

The pre-bathing exercise was not a major physical workout in the manner of the Greek athletes. This was a gentle warm-up prior to bathing. Often the participants would play ball games as part of this routine and five types are mentioned: triple-ball, bladder-ball, handball, feather-ball, and scuffle-ball. Some games were for several players and others were for individuals; they all provided good interest for viewing spectators. Other activities on offer in the larger establishments were boxing, running, wrestling, and fencing. Some of these took place indoors inside large halls built for the purpose. Although swimming was popular in Roman society it was only undertaken to a limited extent in the pools. The baths were not deep, and rarely exceeded 1.0–1.2 metres. Occasionally a pool had a deep end for diving but this was not common. Most baths would have bathers splashing and wading but not swimming seriously. Competitive swimming did take place but it was in rivers, the sea or in specially built gymnasia used exclusively for serious athletic training.

The sequence of bathing activities would begin with the body being anointed with oils, perfumes and cosmetic powders. The mixture plus dirt and dust would then be scraped off with the strigil. At the end of the hot tub the body would again be anointed with oils, expensive perfumes and other unguents. Along with bathing in the hot waters, a patron might retire to the sun-lounge to sun-bathe.

Alongside the routines of cleansing, exercising and bathing, patrons would spend time in leisure and entertainment. This might be chatting and gossiping with friends and family, or it could include poetry reading, music and singing – all by performers both professional and amateur. Larger bathhouses would attract travelling performers such as gymnasts, conjurors, jesters, musicians, singers and mime artists.

Additional to all these activities was of course the need to eat and drink. Food and drink would be available from vendors either inside the bathhouses or from shops and stalls nearby. Descriptions exist of vendors selling cheese, barley, oil, olives, wine, fish, and vegetables; price-lists on the bathhouse wall at Herculaneum note nuts, drinks, hog's fat, bread, meat, and sausage, and the prices of each. Roman bathers ate a lyre-shaped pretzel rather similar to an American bagel. In most cases the patrons were snacking rather than dining – which would be a bigger meal taken later in the day – though archaeological finds of cups, jugs, plates, and the bones of pigs, sheep, and chickens suggest healthy appetites. Patrons were described eating eggs, eels and lettuce in great quantities. Wine was also consumed and sometimes with bad effect. A bather called Philostratus fell down a long flight of steps and died as he left a party at the baths at Sinuessa. The poet Martial observed, 'He would not have incurred such great danger, ye Nymphs, if he had drunk your waters instead.' Martial also noted that a good bath required a good dinner too. 'It is little consolation to bathe in luxury and perish in starvation.' He regarded the dinner or *cena* as the pinnacle of the Roman day.

There is an emphasis on social gatherings for both friendship and for show. Indeed, for the Roman, to dine alone would be indicative of social failure. Furthermore, at the bathhouse and outside it, there would be numerous hangers-on or spongers, all eager to get a free meal and at the expense of a wealthy patron. Martial describes such a social parasite, an individual called Menogenes:

> To escape Menogenes at the warm baths is not possible no matter how hard you try. He will grab the warm hand-ball with right and left so that he can score a point for you. He will pick up the flaccid bladder-ball from the dust for you even if he has already bathed. He'll say your towels are whiter than snow although they may be dirtier than a baby's bib. As you comb your thinning hair he'll say that you have arranged your locks like Achilles ... He'll praise everything, he'll admire everything, until totally exasperated, you will succumb: Come to dinner.

At the same time, the poets might themselves be pursuing a suitable wealthy patron. Martial notes how he had failed to win the attentions of one such individual called Cotta, but another poet, Dento, did. Martial wrote, 'If you wish to feast at Cotta's table, the baths offer the best chance to get an invitation. I never yet dined with him though; my naked charms, I imagine, do not excite his admiration.'

BATHING AND HEALTH

One factor which helped baths and bathing gain so much in popularity in Rome was the deeply entrenched view in many ancient cultures that baths were beneficial for health. From its earliest times, bathing was believed to be curative and preventative in terms of health and disease. Roman and Greek doctors wrote volumes extolling the benefits of various regimes of bathing in hot, cold and lukewarm waters. Bathing at natural hot springs and thermo-mineral baths were believed to be especially effective. Indeed, some of the most popular holiday resorts in Roman times were built around such natural resources. With medicine still very primitive and life-expectancy generally only thirty to thirty-five years or so, the health-giving benefits of water were eagerly sought. Bathing was also to be accompanied by light exercise, for all ages, in the associated gymnasia.

Numerous inscriptions and texts confirm the Roman association of bathing and health. Many of the deities found in bathhouse remains are of those particularly associated with healing and health. Asclepius and Hygieia are two especially common gods of healing. Asclepius was the ancient Greek God of Medicine and Healing and represented the healing aspects of the medical arts. His daughters were Hygieia ('Hygiene'), Iaso ('Medicine'), Aceso ('Healing'), Aglæa ('Healthy Glow'), and Panacea ('Universal Remedy'). Statues might be erected by patrons of the baths or by users keen to ensure the benefits of the healing waters. Inscriptions and other writings stress the links between the baths and health. An advertisement for a bathhouse describes it as 'healthy little baths'.

It is also believed that doctors or physicians may have practiced at the bathhouses. There is no doubt that medical masseurs or *iatraliptae* worked there, and other health-related workers too. Archaeological finds of scalpels and other doctors' instruments in the remains at bathhouses have been taken to indicate that physicians worked there and may even have carried out operations. Of course some of these instruments may have been for cosmetic uses rather than medical ones. There is also evidence that eye doctors practised at the baths and, at least in military facilities, dentists too. It makes sense that physicians might operate to an extent in these surroundings in which their patients came for health-related reasons anyway. A further consideration is that a 'doctor' as we know them today, trained and carefully licensed, is a far cry from those of Roman times. Many physicians would have a smattering of 'science' and a lot of quackery, but hydrotherapy would be something to promote with little risk and a treatment which, if relatively pleasant, would also appeal to the patient. As noted earlier however, some authorities promoted cold-bath treatments in which presumably the healing properties were deemed to be in proportion to the patient's suffering.

Medical training at the time was very limited, and compared with today the health professions were very open to incomers. Essentially anyone who felt like promoting themselves as a doctor could do so. A physician's training was embedded in philosophy rather than any sort of science, and there were no degrees or certificates to provide evidence of experience or competence. Furthermore, there were no systems of monitoring or overseeing the application of medical practice and many people would have some access to aspects of health-related work. Experimentation and experience might lead to some degree of competence and success in dealing with particular ailments, and it is likely then that such knowledge would spread by word of mouth. With much 'popular' medicine and pseudo-medicine disseminated by quacks and conmen, it is likely that anything which seemed to work reasonably well would be a great success. In this context we can understand how hydrotherapy would quickly become popular. First of all the process simply makes you feel good, and secondly, for many minor ailments it would indeed be beneficial. Perhaps too, much was to be made of the 'healing processes' and the fact that patients believed that they were healthier. The pioneering physician Asclepiades (died 91 BC) is credited with triggering much of the subsequent popularity of baths and health-giving places in Rome and then across the Empire. He advocated baths as remedial and preventative measures against illness and disease – hot, dry, wet or cold as appropriate. This advocacy linked to his corpuscular theory of human physiology within which the body was made up of small units and spaces or pores. To maintain or regain health was achieved by getting the correct balance of these units and pores by means of exercise, drink, diet, and of course bathing.

It seems that Asclepiades, from Bythnia (modern-day Turkey), whilst not the only influence on Roman bathing culture, was certainly a key figure. His overall message was that bathing, already available to the wider population of Rome, was both pleasurable but also importantly, it was health-giving. This probably coincided with a trend at the time for Greek and related culture to be fashionable amongst the wealthy ruling elite of Rome. Finally, if we consider the potential threats to human life and health as the great metropolis of Rome grew rapidly around the time of Christ, any help with staying healthy would have been grasped. A possible curative and preventative treatment that could coincide with leisure and pleasure would certainly be popular. As the centuries progressed, the baths became associated with hedonistic pleasures too, and that no doubt sealed their overall success and popularity. Aware of the risks of too much indulgence, physicians and philosophers warned against too much of a good thing.

Over-use of the bathhouse was considered to be a danger to health, and even life-threatening. It was good for you but don't overdo it!

An issue relating to the earlier section on cleanliness and hygiene is the danger of the sick and the healthy all bathing together and in pools with limited sanitation and little or no disinfection. This intimate mixing must have added to the already questionable water quality and the undoubted risks to health. Indeed as the idea of baths was important to Romans for both preventative medicine and curative treatment of illness, the only option open to many sufferers was the public bathhouse. Wealthier citizens would undoubtedly use their own private facilities, but for many it was the public baths or nothing. Writers and others of the time make reference to the sight of the sick at the baths, and to the carrying of illness to such places by the sufferers. One response to this situation was the action taken by Emperor Hadrian when he restricted the use of public baths by the sick to certain hours. This is taken to imply that prior to this measure both sick and healthy bathed together. However, it is unclear how widely the segregation was applied across the Roman provinces. Whereas inscriptions survive from the period demonstrating segregation of male and female bathers, there is no such evidence for the sick. It may be that the regulation was applied only or primarily in Rome, and even then, not to all public baths but just the *thermae* controlled by the Emperor.

There may have been other reasons behind such a move aside from the concerns for public health. One consideration might have been a desire to conceal the unsightly and sick from view in the richly appointed Imperial *thermae*. Since many people suffered – as they did in later medieval times – from unpleasant skin complaints for which they sought cures, this would have been visually disturbing. There seems to be agreement that the sick frequented the public baths. All kinds of illnesses would be on display and as the ideas of bathing and health grew, so then did the number and variety of the sufferers seeking a cure or at least relief. Scribonius Largus described the types and uses of plasters for wound dressing:

> A plaster of indistinct colour is useful for all moderate wounds, animal bites, and contusions or cuts on joints, as when teeth are punched in. Likewise it is remarkably helpful for boils and swellings of the lymphatic glands, completely dissipating hardness as long as it is used for some time. It also draws fluids off long-term ulcer scars and is generally wonderfully good for all sorts of light tasks in daily usage: it doesn't allow tumours or pus to develop; it sticks, so that bandages are unnecessary; and it will not fall off in the bath.

The reference to the bath indicates that the sufferer might well attend such an establishment, and importantly too, that other sorts of bandages and plasters did fall off in such circumstances. In bathing with the sick you would be sharing their open wounds and any seepage, and also an assortment of bandages and plasters that had washed off. Other suggested reasons for restrictions on visiting include a desire to prevent the idle healthy retiring to the bathhouse at times of the day when they should have been gainfully employed.

THERMAL SPAS, SPRINGS AND BATHS

It was possible with Roman technology to artificially heat the bathhouse and the pools. However, some locations had natural thermal springs and became the obvious focus for bathing and curative treatments. Many hot-water springs are also highly sulphurous and this was a property associated with health-giving qualities. A major Italian site was in the volcanic region of Campanula around the Bay of Naples and the major centre of Baiae developed here. The hot-water spas and curative establishments made full use of the abundant hot water and steam. The sources of the hot water and steam were called the 'fields devoured by fire' or the 'Phlegraen Fields' and became hugely popular with visitors. It is believed that the success of the natural hot springs helped make hot-water bathing popular and fashionable in Roman society. The constructed buildings and technology provided a stepping stone to the innovations for artificial heating systems. The public bathhouses that were to emerge represented a coming together of the approaches of traditional Italian domestic farm baths, of the large hot-water mixed bathing pools of the spas, the Greek baths or *balaneia*, and those associated with gymnasia and such establishments.

The natural springs and spas remained hugely popular, perhaps the first major examples of 'health tourism'. Along with the healing properties of locations such as Baiae in the Bay of Naples, the resort was famous for luxury, idleness, wild parties, and drunken orgies both on land and in boats at sea. A more recently discovered 'water-city' is at Allianoi just north-west of Pergamon in modern-day Turkey. This has a grid of streets with extensive visitor facilities, baths, curative places, lodging houses and more.

Sites with hot springs and associated muds would soon become popular, and many have remained so throughout history. Mud baths themselves are ancient treatments rooted in traditions dating back to iconic figures such as Cleopatra, who used mud from the Dead Sea to absorb the natural ingredients from the mud. While these treatments are fun and are used today more for a relaxing and luxurious experience, the practice has actually been used for centuries throughout Europe to treat rheumatism and various skin conditions. Indeed, in a world where understanding of disease and cure was limed, the curative properties of mud applications would be very popular. Disfiguring skin complaints would have been commonplace and were often regarded as leprous, and so any help would have been adopted by the vain or the desperate. The use of naturally occurring mud baths to help with these ailments is known as fangotherapy, and this belongs to the wider spectrum of balneotherapy. Recently (in 2007), a study found that mud baths followed by hot baths can indeed reduce pain and other symptoms in people with fibromyalgia. In this particular case the discovery is an important breakthrough for people suffering from the disease. Interestingly, the findings have not been widely reported; perhaps this is due to the stigma still attached to many medicinal, natural and herbal treatments by the mainstream medical community. People today still use mud baths to treat problems such as arthritis, muscle fatigue, nervous diseases, painful joint diseases, kidney diseases, and urinary infections. Indeed, whilst Western medicine has largely dismissed such treatments as quackery, across Eastern Europe, perhaps a direct descendent of Roman bathing cultures, they are still regarded very highly. Whilst mud baths are often excellent therapeutic treatments for a variety of ailments and diseases, their most popular benefit is on the skin and the complexion. Many people throughout the world swear by mud baths as their fountain of youth. The belief is associated with the chemical make-up with muds containing sulphur, chloride, fluoride and other natural occurring compounds with beneficial properties. In addition, when the mud dries, it also stretches the skin and helps control unsightly wrinkles.

BATHS AND RELIGION

Pre-Christian Roman society involved many personal and household deities, and some specific to particular activities or places. It seems that there was no particular deity for the baths as such. However, many local deities apparently made their homes in springs and wells. In Britain for example, in Roman times, and then later in Medieval times, there were many shrines connected to wells and springs. Coventina's Well on Hadrian's Wall is just one example built probably in the first century AD. Coventina was a Romano-British goddess of wells and springs and is known from multiple inscriptions at one site in Northumberland, in an area surrounding a wellspring near Carrawburgh on Hadrian's Wall. Dedications to Coventina and votive (or religious) offerings were found in a walled area built to contain the outflow from a spring now called 'Coventina's Well'. The well and the walled area surrounding it are close to the site of a Roman fort and settlement on Hadrian's Wall, now known as Carrawburgh. The remains of a Roman *Mithraeum* – a place of worship for the followers of the mystery religion of Mithraism – and a *Nymphaeum* – a monument consecrated to the nymphs and especially those of springs – have also been found near the site. The *Mithraeum* was usually an adapted natural cave or cavern, or a building artificially constructed to mimic a cavern. Even when they were not actually in a subterranean space or in a natural cave, the *Mithraea* were dark and windowless. Wherever possible, the *Mithraea* were in or below an existing building.

It is possible that other inscriptions, two from Hispania and one from Narbonensis, refer to Coventina, but this is apparently uncertain and disputed.

THE CULT AT BATH AND THE ROMAN BATHS

A spring or a well, particularly one with variable or seasonal flow, would be considered to be associated with a powerful deity. This was even more the case if the waters had curative powers. The most striking example of this phenomenon is of course with Aquae Sulis or Bath, in Somerset, in south-west England. The native deity with obvious masculine attributes became identified with Minerva as a goddess, Sulis Minerva. Minerva (from the Etruscan: Menrva), was the Roman goddess, from the second century BC, equated by Romans with the Greek goddess Athena. She was the virgin goddess of poetry, medicine, wisdom, commerce, weaving, crafts and magic, and was often shown with her sacred creature, an owl. This symbolises her ties to wisdom. She was one of three virgin goddesses with Artemis and Hestia, known to Romans as Diana and Vesta.

It seems that Sulis was already the local goddess of the thermal springs that still today feed the spa baths at Bath. These waters were called by the Romans the 'Aquae Sulis' or 'the waters of Sulis'. This retention of the earlier name is not surprising, as Celtic deities often preserved their archaic localisation even when Romanised, associated with a specific place, perhaps a cleft in the earth, a spring, pool, or well. The gilt bronze cult statue of Sulis Minerva was apparently deliberately damaged sometime after the legions departed.

Sulis was therefore a deity worshipped the Romano-British citizens at the thermal spring of Bath, as Sulis Minerva. Her votive objects and inscribed lead tablets suggest that she was seen as both a nourishing, life-giving mother goddess, and usefully as an effective agent of curses wished by her votaries or worshippers. The tablets left at the shrines were often written in code with letters or words written backwards. Word order might also be reversed and lines written in alternating directions, for example, from left to right and then right to left. Most writing from Roman Britain is in Latin; occasionally texts may be in a Celtic language.

Roman culture was of course renowned for its attention to personal cleanliness and hygiene. Any provincial town of note would have built a public bathhouse as a sign of its civilised Romanised nature. As discussed, the general layout of a public bathhouse could be quite elaborate, with separate baths for hot, warm, and cold water, and rooms for exercise. Bathers would, of necessity, leave their clothes and other possessions on pegs or with servants before entering the bath or gymnasium proper. However, despite the watchful eyes of servants or slaves, bathhouses were notorious places for theft. This explains the numerous 'curse tablets' offered to the deities to punish those who stole from them whilst in the bathhouse. Fortuna, the Goddess of Luck, was also associated with bathhouses in recognition of the bathers' vulnerability because they were naked and prey to thieves.

These messages to their deity often relate to theft, perhaps of small amounts of money or clothing taken from the bathhouse. They ask the deity, Sulis Minerva, to punish the known or unknown perpetrators of the crime until they have made effective reparation. A typical example might be that Sulis is asked to affect the physical or mental well-being of the thief. This might be by the prevention of sleep, by stopping normal bodily functions, or even by death. The punishments should only end when the property is returned to the owner, or disposed of as the owner wishes. The latter was often to be its dedication to the deity Sulis. One message found on a tablet in the Temple at Bath has been deciphered as 'Dodimedis has lost two gloves. He asks that the person who has stolen them should lose his mind and eyes in the temple where she appoint.'

The name Sulis has been found almost nowhere other than Bath. However, the goddess is identified with the Suleviae, a group of Celtic goddesses, and they are known to be associated with votive inscriptions in Rome and elsewhere. The link to Suleviae has been confirmed in the epigraphic record from sites at Bath, and the word Suleviae has been suggested as a plural form of Sulis. It is to numerous, mainly widely revered, divine mothers, each having two or three primary aspects to their character. Not all scholars agree on the link and some regard it as purely coincidental. *Suil* in Old Irish is 'eye' or 'gap', and therefore perhaps an entrance to the underworld. However, *Sulis* also means 'sun' and is the original form of current Welsh *haul* (sun), and the Old Irish *suil* (from Indo-European **sawel-*), and Latin *sol* (sun).

The only other British thermal spring is at Buxton and again this was a site known to and occupied by the Romans. Droitwich Spa could perhaps be added, as like Buxton, it is a 'warm' spring. The actual definition of a thermal spring does not necessarily mean that they are very warm. The Institute of Geological Sciences states that it includes 'those waters which at the point of emergence have the same or a greater temperature than the mean average for the surrounding air'. There are or were, nine springs at Buxton and these bring water via the meeting point of Carboniferous Limestone to the south and east, and Millstone Grit to the north and west. The spring-water emerges at a constant temperature of 81.5°F or 27.5°C and has spent around twenty years or more underground since falling as rain on the local catchment. The water has seeped a long way underground to a depth of about 1,800 metres below the limestone. Then, having met a major geological fault in the limestone rocks, the water is squeezed under hydrostatic pressure back to the surface. It emerges with bubbles of gases absorbed into the liquid under pressure deep below the Earth's surface: Nitrogen, Carbon Dioxide, Argon, and Helium. The waters have a high mineral content dominated by Calcium Carbonate from the limestone rocks.

To the Romans, Buxton was known as Aquae Arnemetiae or the 'mineral springs at the sacred grove of the Goddess Arnemetia', the latter being a minor Roman deity. The town lies on the crossing of a number of important Roman roads and was believed to be a retirement or recuperation centre for Roman soldiers from the borders further north. Given the mineral thermal springs, the location would have been of importance to the Romans, although today the details of Roman settlement are elusive. Votive finds of a cache of coins under more modern baths suggest Roman origins, and other archaeological research indicates the presence perhaps of a complex of a Roman Temple and a well plus bathhouse. It has been suggested that there was a mineral spring and a well either on or close to the modern 'Natural Baths', and a larger bathhouse now buried beneath the former St Ann's Hotel at the western end of the famous Georgian Crescent. The hotel closed in the latter part of the twentieth century as the building was in need of major repairs.

MILITARY BATHHOUSES

Other deities were also to be found at Roman baths. For example, with military baths it was common to include altars to Fortuna or figures of Fortuna, the Roman goddess of Fortune. She was the goddess who protected men when at their most vulnerable, and in this case, when they were naked. Such an altar to Fortuna was found at the bathhouse in Chesters in Northumbria. Fortuna was the Roman goddess and the equivalent of the Greek goddess Tyche. She was the bringer of fortune and the personification of luck, good or bad, in Roman religion. Represented as veiled and blind, like in modern depictions of Justice, she represented fate.

Fortuna Balnearis, meaning 'Fortuna of the Baths', was the manifestation of the Roman Goddess of Fortune associated with bathhouses as a Goddess of Health as well as good luck. She was particularly the subject of worship by soldiers in remote outposts such as in Britain. Other manifestations of Fortuna included Fortuna Salutaris ('Wholesome' and 'Health-bringing Fortuna') and Fortuna Redux ('Fortuna Who Brings [Soldiers] Home'). These dedications reflect the concerns of individuals situated far from their homeland and often in hostile, unwelcoming territories. Fortuna Balnearis was particularly a Goddess of military bathhouses, and reflected the additional uncertainties and vulnerabilities of frontier soldiers. The goddess's aspects of *salutaris* and *redux* concerned both health and returning home safely. It is likely that Fortuna Balnearis was also concerned with soldiers' health, and especially the practice of good hygiene and exercise – things that would have separated the Romans from their uncivilised hosts.

The commandant's quarters generally included private rooms and at least a private toilet. Sometimes, but not always, they included private baths. In many cases the commanding officer had to join his troops in the garrison bathhouse, which until the times of the late Empire, around AD 400–500, were almost always outside the fort walls. Most forts, even small ones, would have a degree of hygiene in terms of toilets that was unparalleled until the twentieth century. Close to the ramparts would be latrines with wooden seats over stone-built flushed sewers. Sponges were provided in place of modern-day toilet paper, and were rinsed in the running water of the gulley below (although this of course would be carrying the waste from other latrine users!). Tubs of water were provided to wash the hands prior to leave the facility. Water-tanks were positioned around the garrison walls to collect rainwater for washing and for drinking. With a garrison of hundreds of men the latrines and their sewers required constant flushing to avoid dirt and disease. As noted, some water was collected in rainwater tanks, but to flush out the sewers necessitated running water in good supply, so local streams were diverted to this end. Open channel aqueducts carried running water from nearby streams to the forts; that at Greatchester on Hadrian's Wall, for example, was around 8 km long.

In the provinces, it seems that military bathhouses were generally outside the fortification and they varied greatly in both size and their degree of complexity. This location may be because the baths were to an extent outside direct military discipline, and because the locality was considered to be safe. In forts along the Antonine Wall for example, the bathhouse is sometimes within the protected area, mostly tucked away inside a corner of the protective wall. There is also evidence of them being used for mixed bathing or, at least at times, for women bathers. The drains or such facilities frequently turn up archaeological finds of hairpins, broaches, and other jewellery which indicate female usage from the *vicus* or neighbourhood. In many military locations the bathhouse is the most significant built structure outside of the fort walls. Essential to the mental and physical health and well-being of the soldiers, the baths were a prestigious building. They would stand out from the rather basic buildings of local native people that clustered around every settlement. These would be rough timber frame buildings to house all the folk drawn to a fort and its garrison of, say, 500 soldiers, its merchants and tradesmen, and the service sector of taverns, gambling houses, and brothels.

THE BATHERS

Who used the baths – and where and when they did so – varied through time with social norms and with whether the baths were public or private. In the latter cases, it is likely that the whole family might bathe together. Slaves and servants would be in attendance in both private and public facilities, in providing the bathhouse service and in attending to their masters and mistresses. Personal slaves would accompany the bather and help with undressing and dressing, and with applying the strigil. It is reputed that when in northern Britain, Hadrian witnessed a man scraping his back on the famous wall, no servant in attendance. The Emperor therefore gave the man a slave to apply the strigil for him. The next time he visited the same spot, there were many old men all scraping their backs on the masonry; so Hadrian gave them all strigils and told them to scrape each other.

There is also the vexed question of whether for example slaves were allowed to bathe. However, it seems that this depended on the enlightenment of the master. The most important writer on Roman agriculture, Lucius Columella (died AD 70), stated, 'It is important that there should be such places in which the servants may bathe – but only on holidays, for frequent bathing is not conducive to physical vigour.'

Many villas do appear to have two sets of baths, perhaps one for the master and his family, and the other for the steward, and/or for slaves or servants. Another explanation is that these are simply baths built and used during different periods, rather than being contemporary.

4

LEISURE, ROME & DECADENCE

An immediate and obvious question for anyone considering Roman baths and bathing is why they were so popular and so important. Bathing became an important part of Roman culture, of being 'Roman'. The visit to the bathhouse became a vital part of the Roman daily habit, in effect a ritual, and it became deeply ingrained in Roman culture. The Roman day had the afternoon set aside for leisure. The workday would have begun early and they worked hard through the morning. Then the emphasis of the day moved on to social and leisure activities. Having a light lunch followed by a siesta in the public baths had become an important and enjoyable part of Roman life as early as the end of the Republic. This was a comforting part of civilised urban living and thus an important part of being 'Roman'. Martial recommended the eighth hour as the best for bathing since 'this hour tempers the warm baths …'

In considering the great bathhouses such as the *thermae* one wonders what it was like to experience this uniquely luxurious leisurely activity. How did the ordinary bathers feel before, during and after their immersion? One bath-side inscription begins 'wonder seizes me …' and follows with a lavish description of the bathing environment, with its marble-clad walls, gold ceilings, and rich adornments in every room. These were opulent showcases for luxurious living. There were undoubtedly small, grubby, dingy baths as well, but we tend to hear less about those. The *thermae* were large, open, spacious, and splendid, with ceilings maybe up to 30–40 metres high. In the context of the time, these are massive structures and they were richly adorned with sculptures, paintings, mosaics and other ornaments. Combined with the heat, humidity and fragrance of oils and perfumes, the whole experience would be heavily sensual. Noise from the various activities would echo within and between rooms and add to the heady atmosphere of the place.

Most bathing took place during daylight hours though there is evidence of artificial lighting with oil lamps at some baths. Indeed, most public baths were closed by Imperial decree before darkness fell. Some night-time bathing did take place and the Emperor Alexander Severus (AD 208–35) 'donated oil for the lighting of the baths'. These had previously been closed before sunset, and one reason was to avoid night-time disturbances. Most bathhouses closed at sunset but after this time, whilst the sober and conservative citizen might return home to dine, the pleasure-seeker would find much on offer. Besides the circus and the amphitheatre, there were abundant brothels outside which the prostitutes would display themselves on benches. These included many foreign women, Egyptian and Syrian, wearing dramatically bright clothes that marked them out from 'respectable' women. They had short tunics or togas and bangles around their ankles. However, despite society views today, the prostitutes were an accepted part of Roman urban culture and were organised and taxed on the basis of the fees they charged their customers. They were allowed to parade in the streets and in Rome itself, they were a common sight along the Via Sacra and in the Subura, and were considered to be an important part of the city economy. This bustling, noisy, crowded part of the City of Rome was described by Juvenal as the 'boiling Subura' and was where the adventurous pleasure-seekers might head after the bathhouses closed. Indeed, to be seen at least occasionally as associating with a prostitute in these quarters was not considered unusual or reprehensible for a young man of a good upbringing. There was some knowledge of the possible dangers of venereal disease but that was not yet a serious problem. Like the bathhouses, the hours of opening of the brothels were regulated by the State, but those of the taverns were not. Gambling was also rife and despite attempts at regulation, was not controlled. So, even when the baths closed for the night there was plenty more that the Roman or Romanised populations might enjoy.

Bathing was – and indeed is – a highly pleasurable experience. It is physically and psychologically enjoyable to have warm, moist air and water on or around the body, and to experience this with pleasant, sometimes opulent surroundings and massage was highly satisfying. This relaxation with warm and clean(ish) water, oils and perfumes, and with smooth marble surfaces, richly decorated plasterwork, good food and drink, was the means to the Roman state of enjoyment called *voluptas*. Furthermore, this sensuous and healthy experience could be had communally so a whole group of family, friends and acquaintances might bathe and relax together. The soporific warmth and humidity of the pools and the fragrant oils and perfumes combined to create a world of classless nakedness that encouraged intimacy and friendship. Throughout much of the Roman period, though by no means for everyone or for the entire time, mixed nude bathing was also the custom.

In the sumptuous and lavish surroundings of the great public baths, the imperial *thermae* the sense of pleasure, leisure and sensuous delight would have been overwhelming. With wonderful coloured marbles, richly decorated mosaics, ornamental plasterwork, fine statues and bronze hardware, the bather could relax and enjoy. The whole experience was presented under grand vaults and domes with abundant lighting and a lofty elegance. It is this voluptuous pinnacle of civilisation that was captured in the writings of poets such as Martial, a writer in the first century. Another poet, Statius, wrote of the luxurious Baths of Etruscus in Rome: 'Toil and care, depart! I sing of the baths that sparkle with bright marbles! ... Come, then, ye nymphs of the waters, turn your clean faces and bind up your glass-green hair with tender wine shoots, your naked bodies as you emerge from the deep springs, and torture your satyr-lovers with the sight!' He was describing the mythical creatures which inhabited the natural springs of the hills of Rome and mingled with the waters of the great aqueducts. These particular waters which fed the Baths of Etruscus were especially pure and excellent for swimming and bathing.

The baths were meeting places for society and politicians, and places for leisure, recreation and often for decadent excess. It is suggested that the way that Romans used their baths was a matter of personal taste, fashion and medical advice. The particular conditions available and treatments on offer would likewise vary. For example, there were regimes of usage prescribed fro the sick and the infirm. However, as has been the case throughout history there was much debate and disagreement about the uses and misuses of bathing. Baths and bathing have always been associated with a degree of mystique and quackery, and apparently, it was the same in Roman times.

At the bathing suites of a private domestic household, the users would change in the cool room and then probably progress to the warm dry room where oils would be applied to the body. They would then move to the hot steamy room to encourage sweating and here they would be scraped with the strigil to remove oil and dirt. Following this, the bather would progress to a hot bath and finally would return to the cool room to be washed and cooled with cold water. Larger facilities such as public baths and military establishments sometimes also offered a hot dry room.

The balance between utility and decadence or pleasure in the baths was always difficult. Seneca contrasted the values and styles or fashions of an older generation with those of his own day:

> We think ourselves poor and mean if our walls are not resplendent with large and costly mirrors; if our marbles [decorating our baths] from faraway Alexandria are not set off by mosaics of rich, yellow stone from Numidia … If our vaulted ceilings are not buried in glass; if our swimming pools are not lined with marble from Thasos, once a rare and wonderful sight in any temple … and finally, if water is not poured from silver faucets … What a vast number of statues, of columns that support nothing but are built for mere decoration, merely in order to spend more money! And what masses of water fall crashing from level to level! We have become so luxurious that we have nothing but precious stones to walk upon.

Seneca may be exaggerating for effect, but only a little. The evidence we have is that many Italian bathhouses were indeed splendidly and expensively furnished and decorated. He goes on to contrast the highly lit baths of his time with the dark and dingy structures of earlier less pleasure-seeking generations:

> For our ancestors did not think that one could have a hot bath except in darkness … nowadays, however, people regard baths as fit only for moths if they have not been arranged so that they receive the sun all day long through largest of windows, if men cannot look out from their bath-tubs over stretches of land and sea.

Seneca was perhaps giving an old-fashioned criticism of the modern trends. He disapproved of the luxurious and even decadent lifestyles developing in the Empire in contrast to the frugal and military virtues so favoured in earlier times. He regretted 'even the popular habit of bathing every day, instead of once a week as the old Romans such as Scipio, used to do … Now that the spick-and-span bathing establishments have been devised, men are really fouler than of yore.' He was writing for a disapproving audience concerned about moral decline and this was encapsulated by the luxurious and, in their views, wasteful decadence of the bathhouses. This opinion condemned the moral decay and the sexual licentiousness that were, they felt, encouraged by the baths, and which flourished in this environment. Indeed, this was ultimately to be the basis of Christian disapproval of bathing and the major cause of its decline in the post-Roman centuries.

One of Seneca's contemporaries was a philosopher called Demetrius the Cynic. At the dedication of the Thermae of Nero in Rome, he reputedly spoke out against 'people who bathed, declaring that bathing enfeebled and polluted one; and declared that such institutions were a useless expense.' According to Yegül (2010) Demetrius was lucky to escape with his life. This was not a time or indeed an audience suited to such direct criticism.

Pliny the Elder was another writer of the time. He wrote of the issues of excessive anointing and bathing as grim indicators of a spreading social disease (Yegül, 2010). He went on to describe 'the broiling baths by which they have persuade us that food is cooked in our bodies so that everybody leaves them weaker for treatment and the most submissive are carried out to be buried'. In a humorous quip, Pliny suggested that a slave condemned for some criminal offence should be 'bathed alive', and he wrote of how the 'fashionable heat' of the baths was a proper conflagration.

Whatever the opinions and the criticisms of the day, the baths were ever-popular and increasingly frequented. This aspect of Roman culture affected everyone, every class, and every society across a vast empire. Great emperors lived in and amongst their baths and banquets in resplendent imperial palaces. Commodus, an emperor in the second century AD, was reputed to bathe seven or eight times a day.

DECADENCE AND ANTI-SOCIAL BEHAVIOUR

Conservative writers and philosophers raged at the moves to what they saw as licentiousness and uncivilised or uncouth behaviour. Certainly the splendid bathhouses provided abundant opportunities for the rich to display their wealth and the vain to show off in petty and annoying ways. The mixed culture of the bathhouses also provided chance for the more lowly to be loutish and boorish. Wealthy young men would show off with expensive and lavish jewellery, or display their naked bodies to crowds of applauding admirers. Recitals of amateur and often vulgar poetry caused amusement and offence, probably in equal portions. This was not necessarily a new phenomenon, and indeed Horace, a poet of the late Republic, had commented on such behaviour in earlier times. 'Many there are who recite their writings in the middle of the Forum, or in the baths. How pleasantly the vaulted space echoes the voice! That delights the fools who never ask themselves whether what they do is in bad taste or out of season.'

Martial chips in with his own views on amateur recitals: 'You read to me as I stand, you read to me as I sit. You read to me as I run, you read to me as

I shit. I escape to the baths; you buzz my ear. I head for the pool; I am not allowed to swim. I haste for dinner, you stop me as I go. I reach the table, you drive me away as I eat.'

There could also be violence and unrest at the baths. One Macedo died following a beating from his own slaves after which they threw him onto the scalding hot floor of his private bath. He recovered consciousness but died some days later. He had already been the victim of violence at the public bathhouse when he was punched, this time through a case of mistaken identity; perhaps he was just unlucky.

Although the bathhouse was intended to be a place of health and fitness, as a centre of leisure activities it became a focus for over-indulgence. In particular, and as noted by the disapproving Seneca, they were the cause of eating and drinking to excess. He describes this as one of youth's popular vices. The idea was to build up strength by exercise in order to then drink around the baths amongst naked bathers; even to bathe in wine and to rub off the sweat caused by excessive drinking. In particular, the sweat chambers were used to stimulate a great thirst. Pliny the Elder wrote, 'actually, unable to wait to get home to dinner! No, not even to put their clothes on, but on the spot, while still naked, they lift up huge vessels [of wine] as if to show off their strength, and pour down the whole contents, then raise it up again, to take another swig.' Others commented on how bathhouse patrons didn't know how to get home sober.

The bathhouse was certainly an outlet for excessive behaviour; yet gluttony and overindulgence were widely disapproved of. The objections were both social disapproval and genuine concerns over health. The dangers of bathing on a full stomach or after excessive wine were widely recognised. Many when bathing, and certainly the older and frailer members of society, would eat very frugally – simply for the sake of their health. From the writers of the time, it is suggested that often it was the newly-rich and the young who were most likely to overindulge. Juvenal, a satirist of the second century AD wrote, 'But you will pay the price all too soon, my friend, when you undress and waddle into your bath, your belly swollen with undigested peacock meat – a lightning heart attack with no time to make your will.'

SEX AND NUDITY IN THE BATHS

It is hard to separate reality from myth in the history of the Roman baths. Above all, the idea of the baths as centres for nudity and licentious behaviour has captured the imaginations of people from that time to the present day. The thermo-mineral spas such as Baiae in the Bay of Naples became famous and synonymous with unrestrained sex and sensual, dissolute activities. Martial wrote of his friend Laevinia who was transformed from a dutiful and sober wife at home to a wild and sensual creature by a visit to the thermal spa at Baiae. She ran off with a younger man. Clearly the mixing of the sexes, the leisurely atmosphere with good food, wine and recreational pursuits, and the bathing and nudity created an all-pervading sensual experience. Even the often prudish Victorians were able to use 'artistic representations of such classical scenes' as an excuse to paint naked ladies. How much of this is truth and how much is myth is difficult to discern. The baths certainly provided the opportunity to see and to be seen, and nudity was accepted and commonplace here. Skimpy costumes worn during initial oiling and massage, or in the sweat tub, would certainly be cast off when it came to bathing with full immersion. This may have been something that was very normal and part of the bathing routine, and not necessarily sensual or sexual. It may be that both situations occurred depending on the time and the place. Contemporary paintings from a bathhouse in the second century AD give the impression of Roman ladies bathing nude and at their toilette, but are not sexually charged. A simple bathing wrap may have provided a token of modesty and restraint. Certainly in some social circles, full nudity at the baths would have caused offence. In more old-fashioned and conservative families it was even advised that fathers should not bathe with their grown-up sons or with their sons-in-law 'because they were ashamed to uncover their nakedness'. Phryne, a famous and beautiful courtesan posed naked for the painter Apelles in a painting of Aphrodite, but she was too shy to go to the public baths. Not all Roman ladies were so bashful, and Martial writes of his exchange with a lady called Galla: 'When I compliment your face, when I admire your legs and hands, you are accustomed to say, "Naked I please you more, yet, you continually avoid taking a bath with me. Surely you are not afraid, Galla, that I shall not please you."'

Writers of the time make it clear that men and women, married and unmarried, could and would bathe together in the nude and this did not necessarily imply impropriety. Intimate behaviour could take place without the suggestion of adultery. However, Pliny the Elder still cited mixed nude bathing as one of the undesirable manifestations of the new decadence. The poet Martial on the other hand, writing at a later date, makes it clear that for him at any rate, mixed nude bathing was the norm. Whether this reflects social norms or Martial's particular and personal tastes is a matter for conjecture. On balance, it is likely that conservative Roman society viewed such behaviour as on the edge of decency and somewhat hedonistic. What the majority of the Roman public thought or felt is hard to determine. There is plenty of evidence that respectable women, mothers, and others did visit the baths and would bathe nude either in single-sex sessions or mixed with men, and this was a routine pleasurable activity with no hint of inappropriate behaviour. However, whilst this was certainly the case, there is plenty of evidence too, that demonstrates that the bathhouse was very much a focus for other more permissive activities. There are abundant references which testify to the baths being frequented by courtesans and by prostitutes of both sexes. Taking a bath with a courtesan was the natural prelude to other intimacies. As noted earlier, the two slaves Dexter and Apelles were recorded as having sexual relations with women at a bathhouse in Herculaneum. The explicit graffiti states that 'Apelles the Mouse with his brother Dexter lovingly fucked two women twice'. As Yegül (2010) points out, this is unequivocal evidence of a pretty sordid affair.

Further evidence or indication of the activities which went on at the baths is the bathing parties that could be arranged for rich patrons. In a play by Plautus, a second-century-BC writer, a pimp tries to draw a wealthy man called Collymore into the bathhouse in order to participate in the pleasures of 'a nicely cushioned couch with a nice lady to love' and then a 'love-bath' with abundant wine. The poet Ovid suggests the baths as a good place to meet your lovers. He wrote, 'What is the use of guarding women ... when while the guardian keeps the girl's clothes outside the baths, hidden lovers lurk safely within?' Furthermore, in visiting the baths you were able to sweat out the effects of earlier overindulgence and begin anew.

As discussed earlier, one approach adopted was to segregate male and female bathing either into different baths, or at least by different times. This was not always easy to enforce, and sometimes the intervention of the gods was required. One inscription found by archaeologists at a small bathhouse in Trastevere in Rome stated, 'By order of the almighty god Silvanus, women are prohibited from stepping into the swimming pool reserved for men.' The scholar who found the inscription noted that 'This inscription shows that police regulations were not enough to keep fast women in order ... the owners of the baths were obliged to resort to the intervention of the gods.'

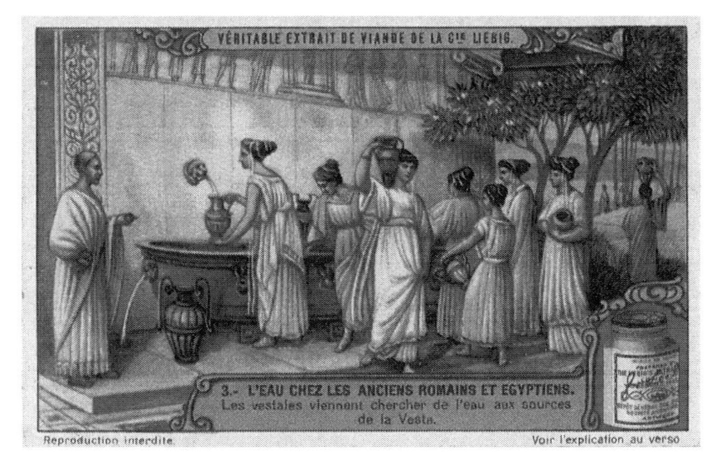

1 Advertising card showing Roman slaves collecting water.

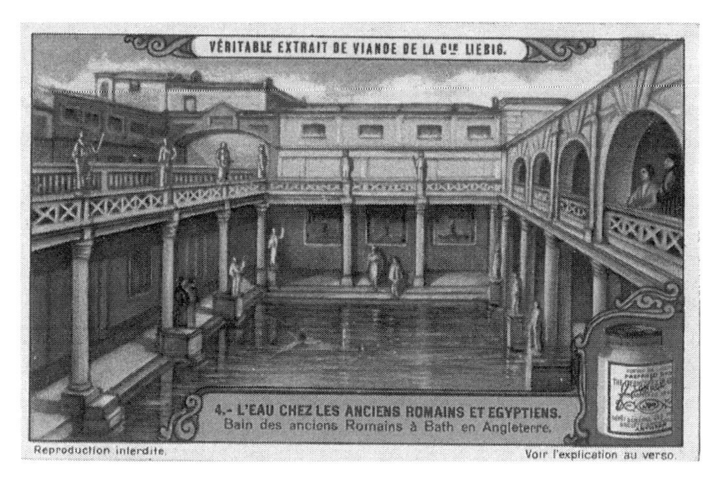

2 Advertising card showing the Roman Baths at Bath.

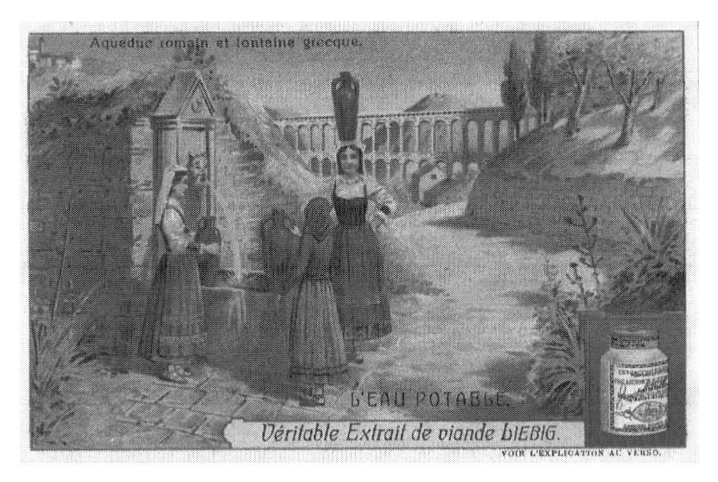

3 Advertising card showing the spring and well.

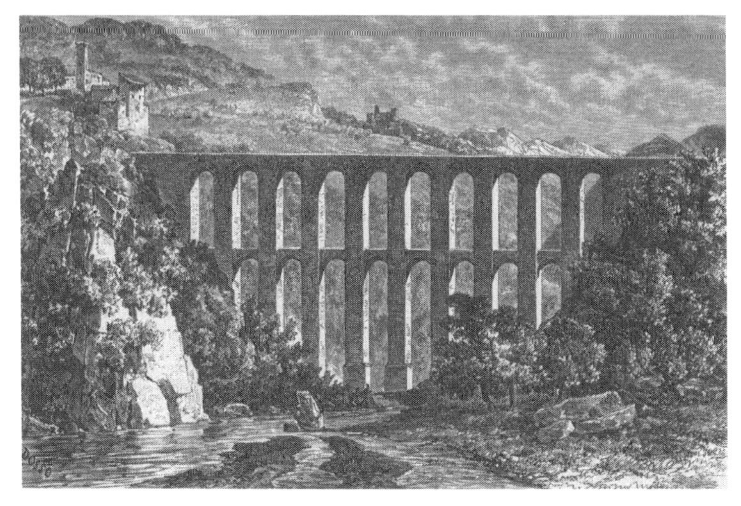

4 Aqueduct of Spoleto.

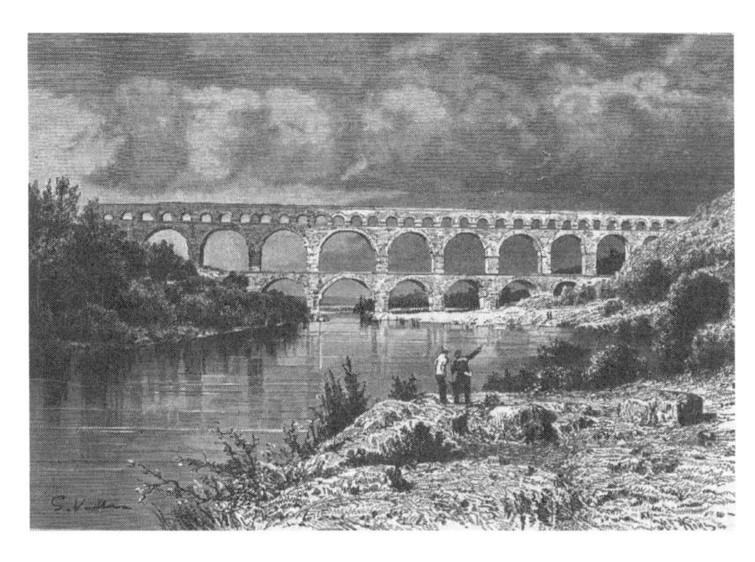

5 Pont du Gard Roman aqueduct at Nimes.

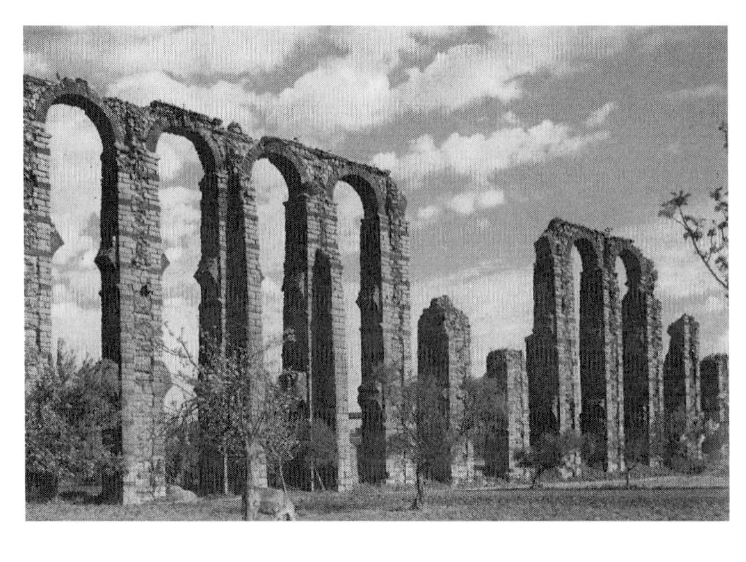

6 Roman aqueduct, Merida, 1970s.

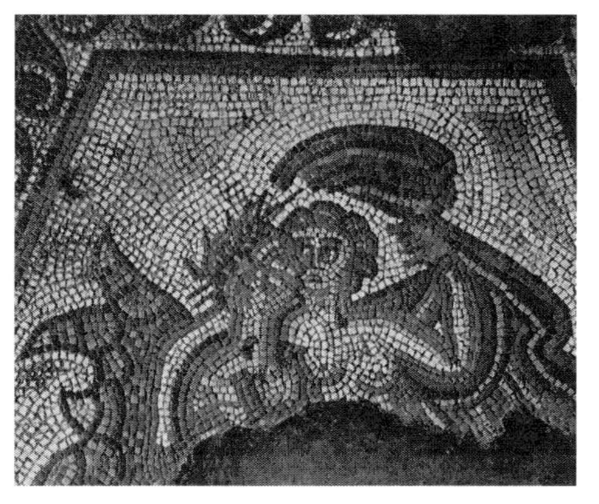

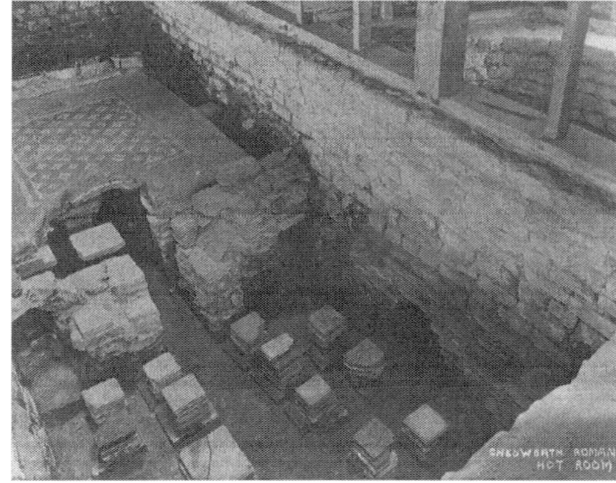

Above left: 7 Mosaic, Chedworth Villa.

Above right: 8 Chedworth Roman Villa bathhouse hot room.

Below: 9 Hypocaust at the Roman Baths in Bath. (© Bath & North East Somerset Council)

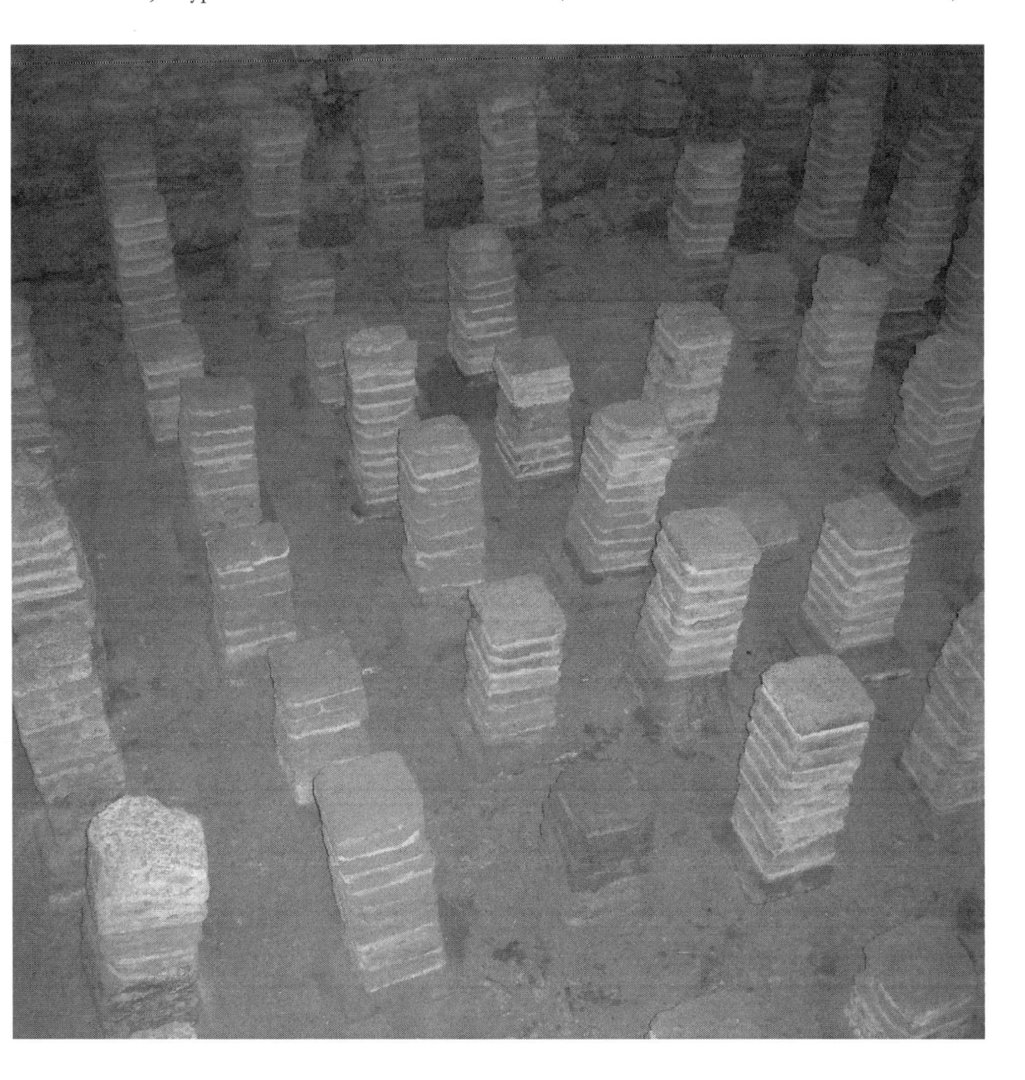

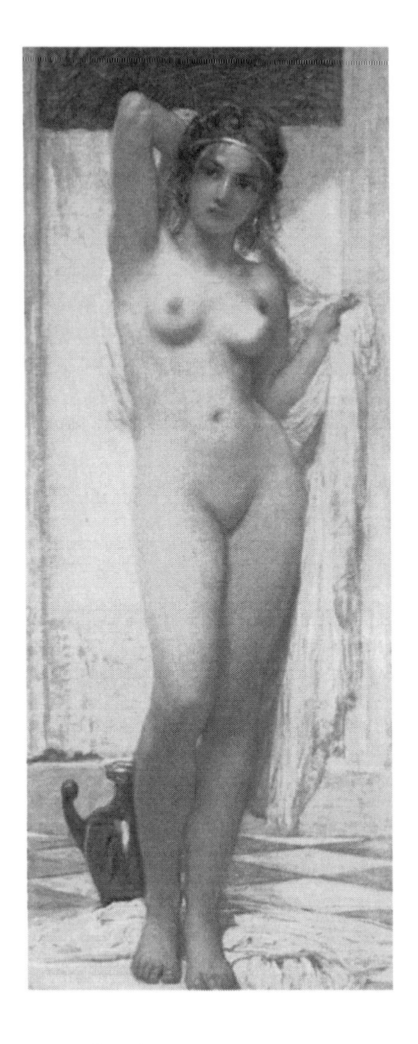

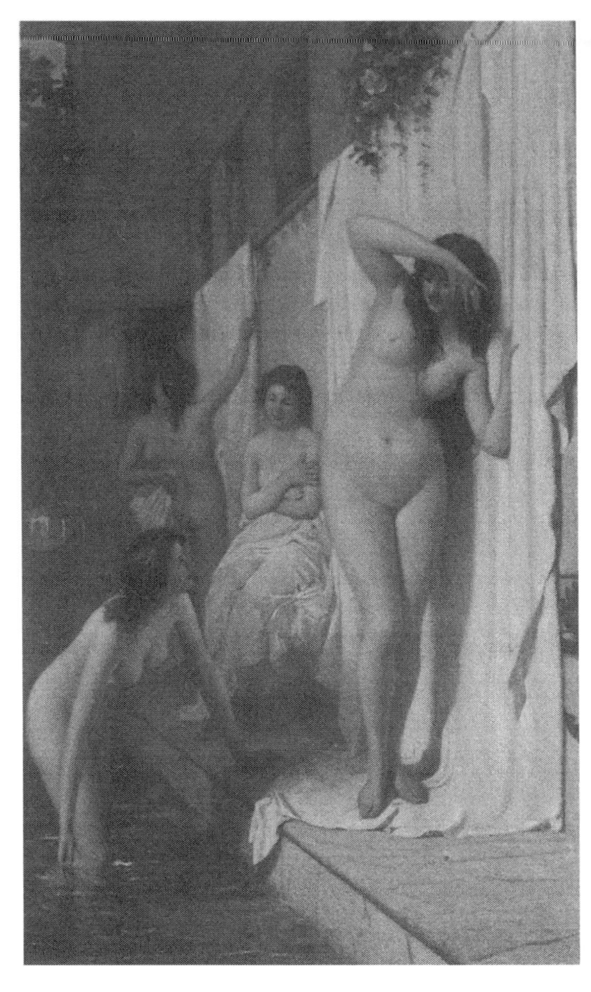

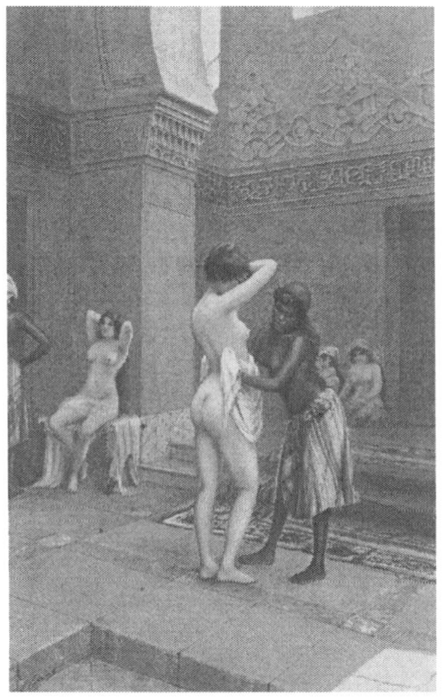

Above left: 10 Roman woman bathing by Karoly Lotz.

Above right: 11 Roman women at the Pompeii Bathhouse.

Left: 12 Roman women bathers attended by slaves.

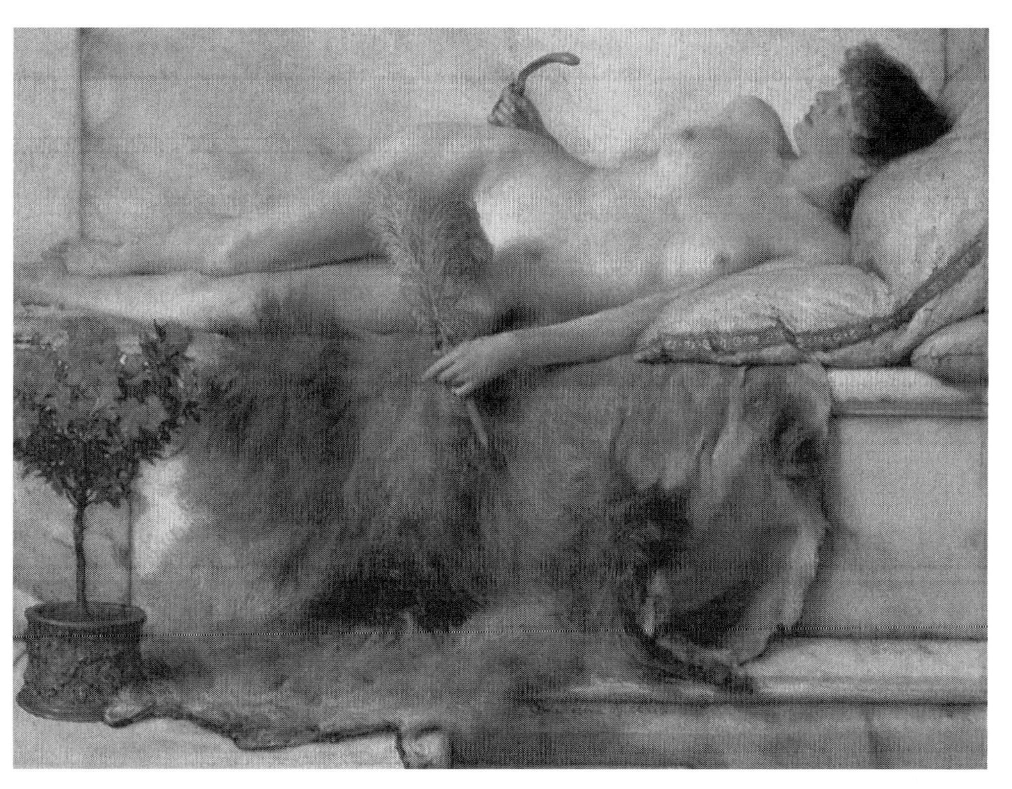

13 Roman woman with strigil by Sir Lawrence Alma-Tadema.

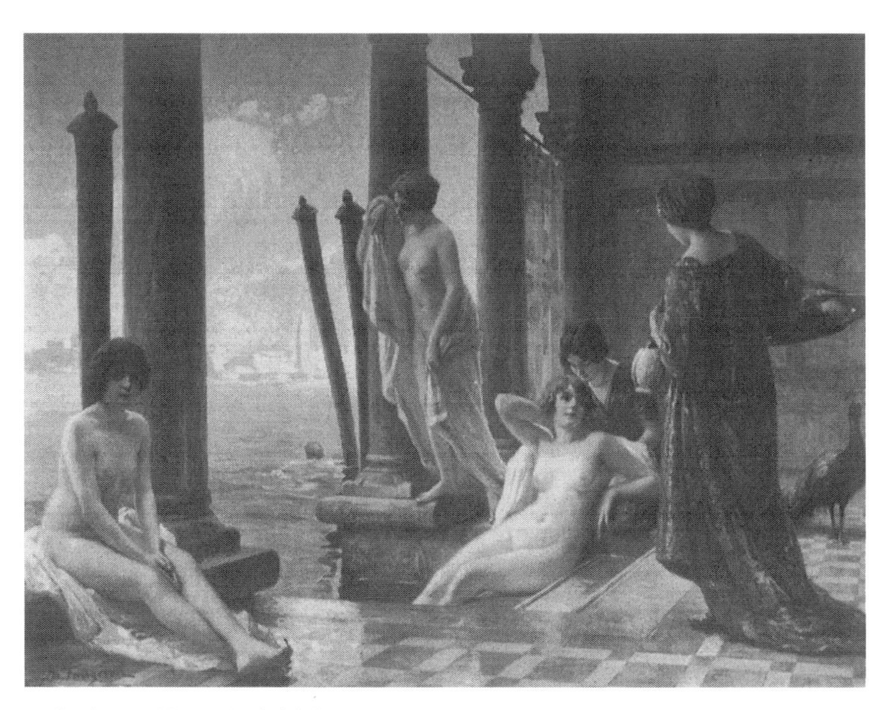

14 Bathers at Venice by Adolphe Faugeron.

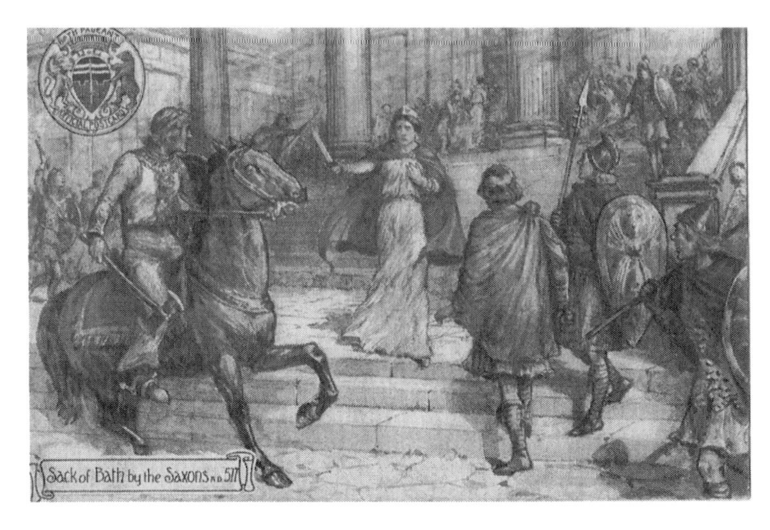

15 The sack of Bath by the Saxons.

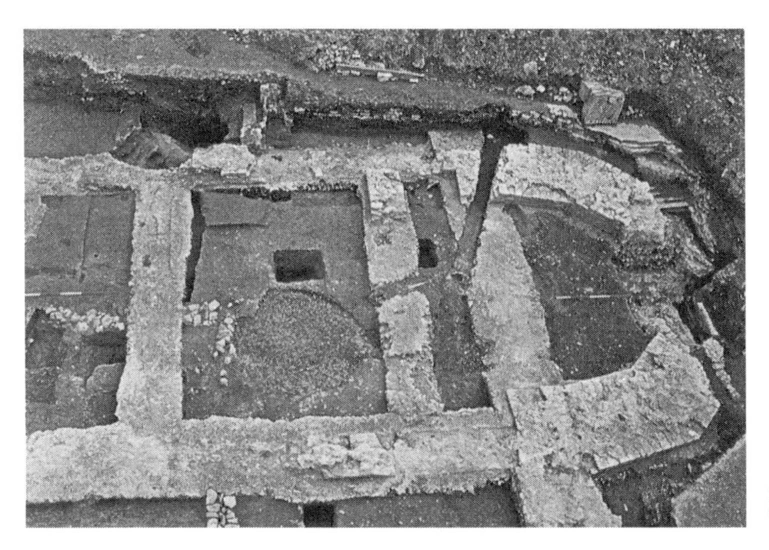

16 Roman ruins, York, 1970s.

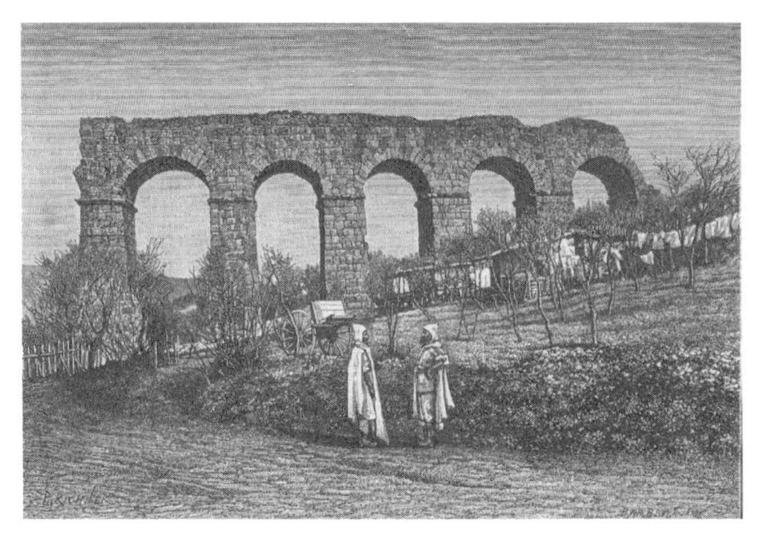

17 Ruins of a Roman aqueduct near Constantine.

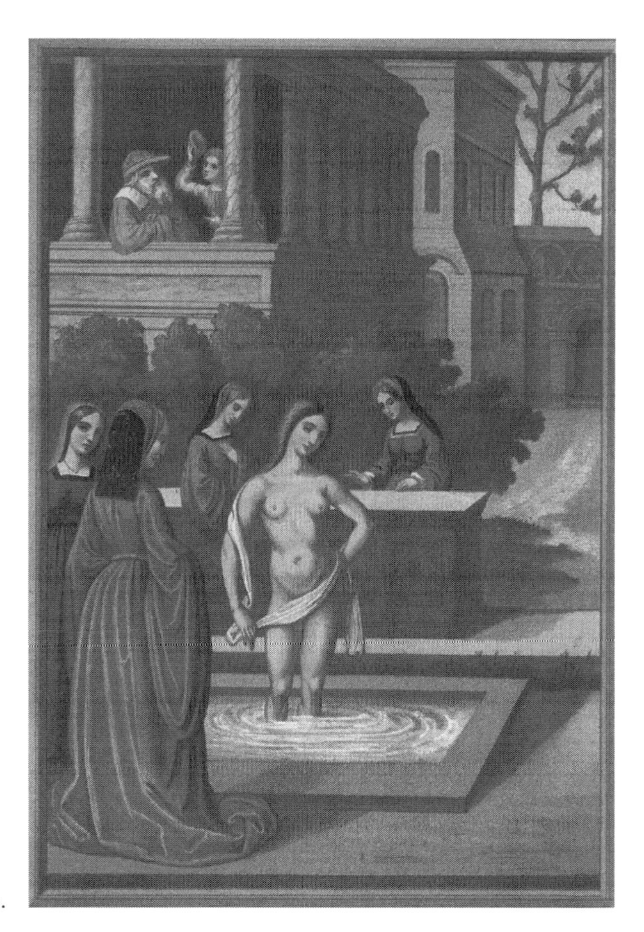

18 Medieval bathing scene.

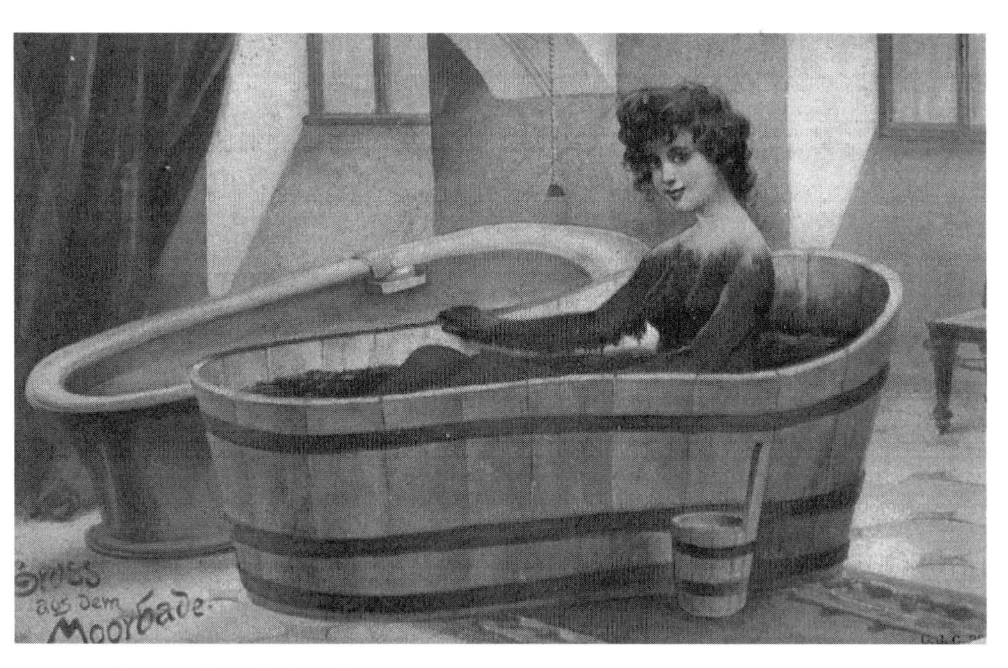

19 German Moor Bath, early 1900s.

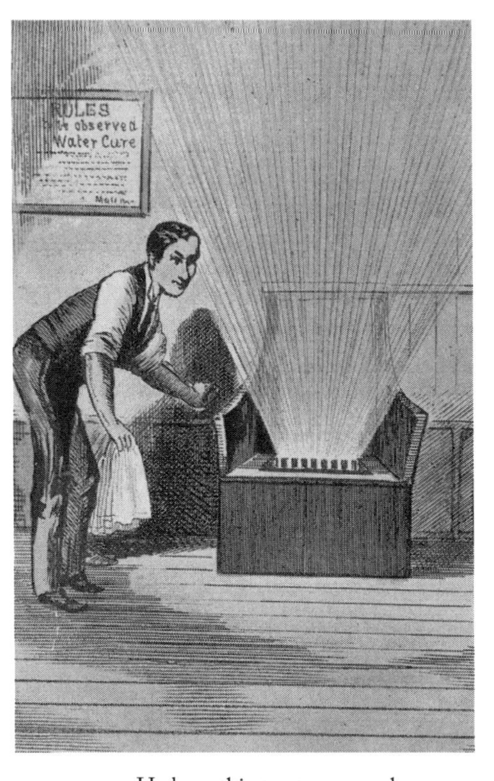

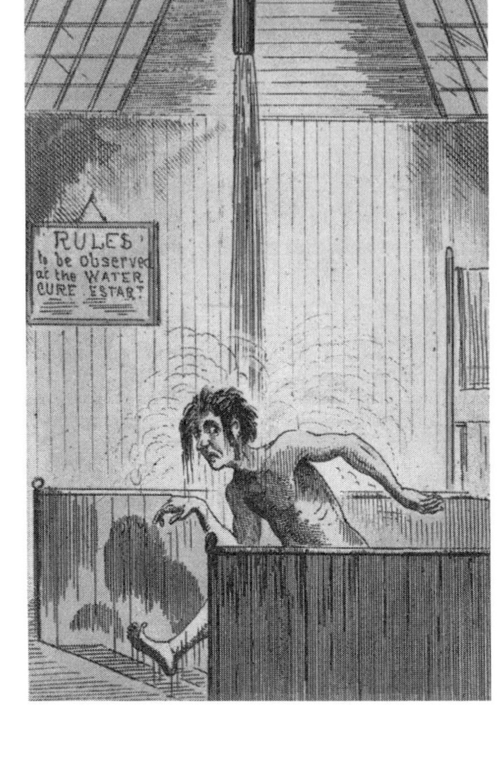

20, 21, 22, 23 Hydropathic treatment, early 1900s.

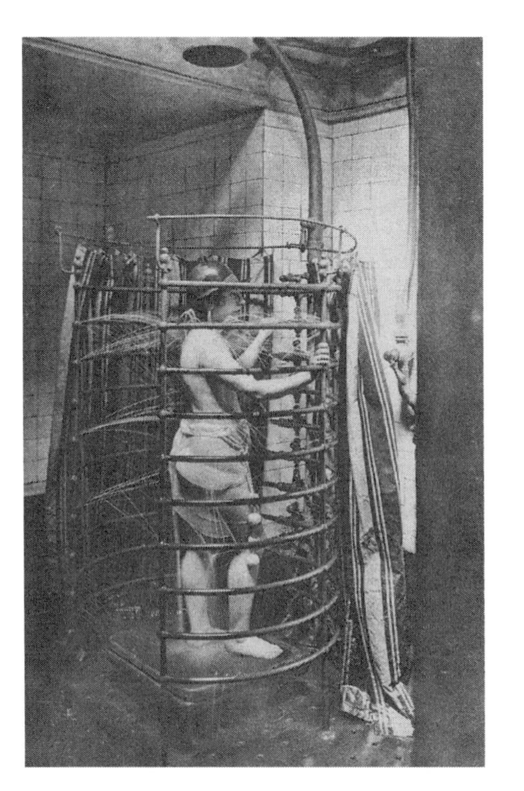

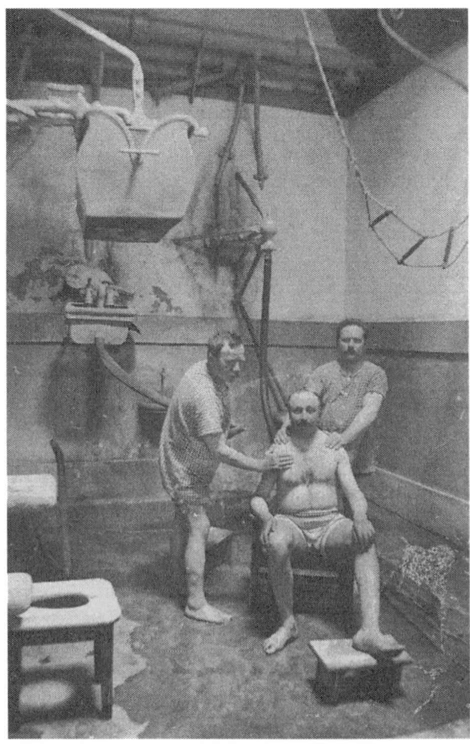

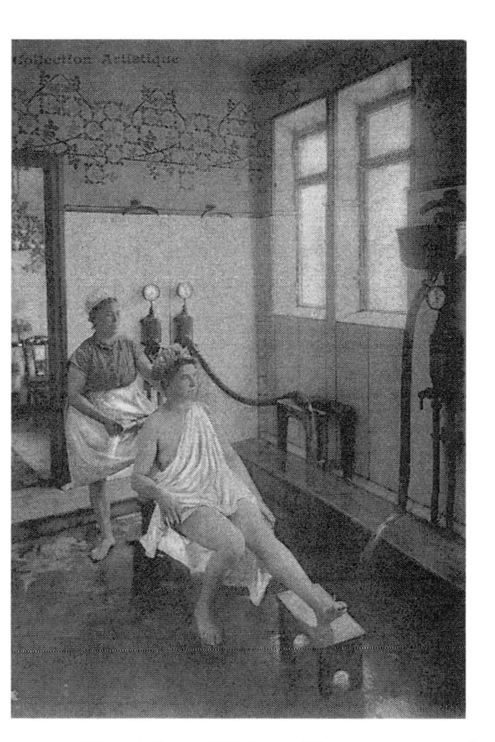

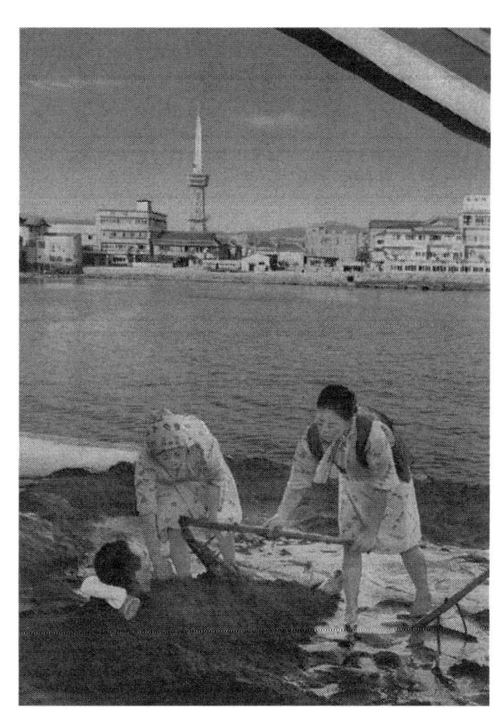

Above left: 24 Hydropathic treatment, early 1900s.

Above right: 25 Taking a hot sand bath, Sunayu, Japan, 1960s.

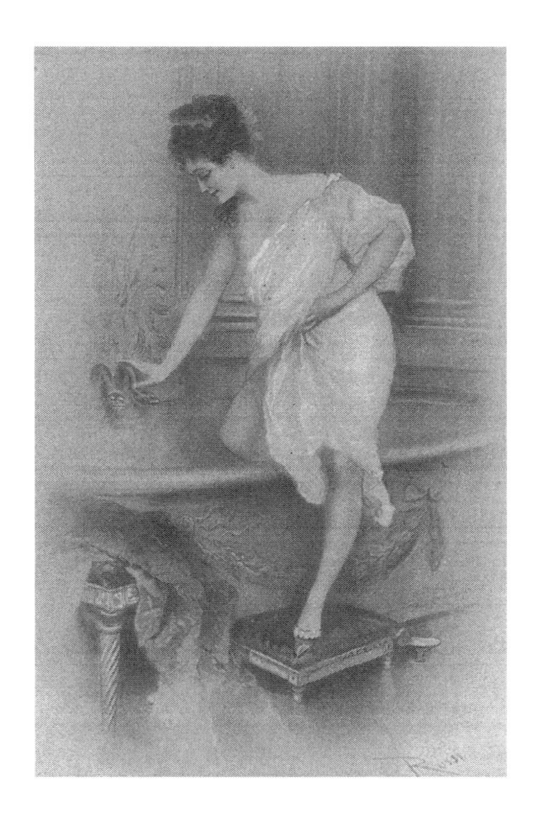

26 Bathing, 1903.

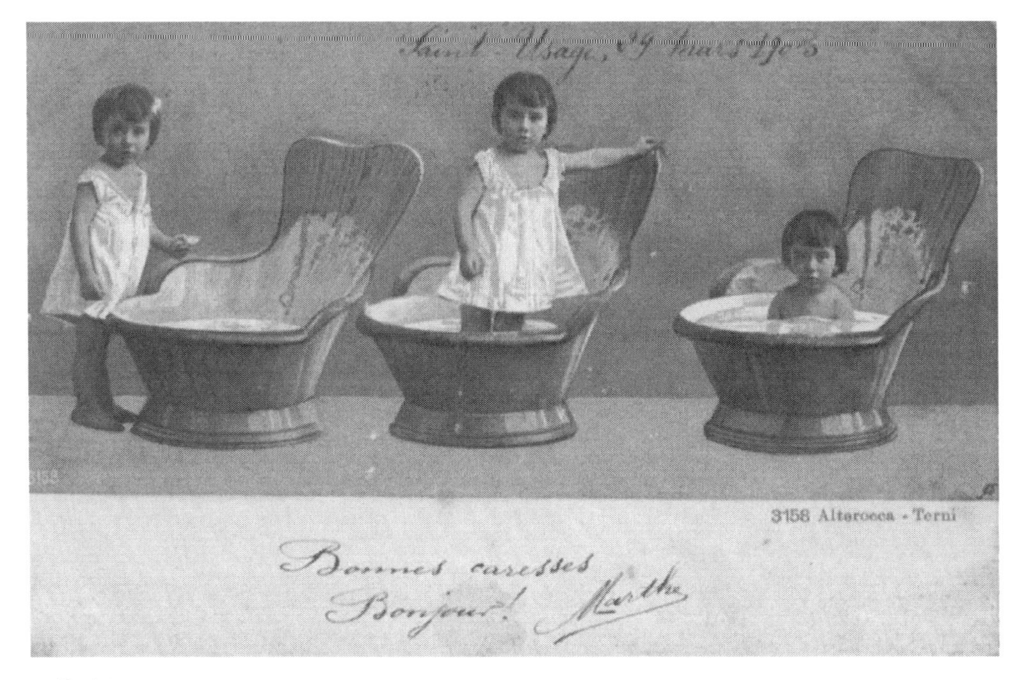

27 Bathing, 1906.

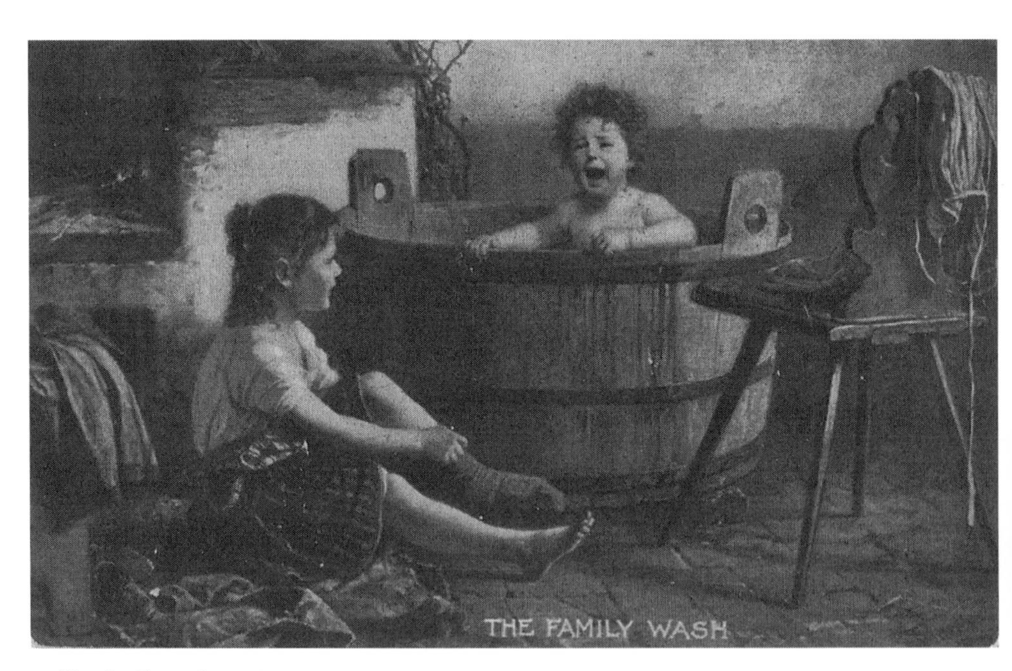

28 The family wash, 1908.

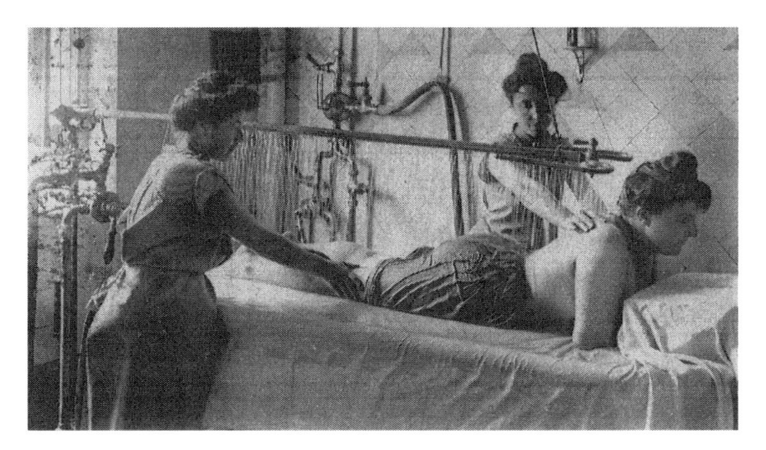

29 Treatment at the Vichy Thermal Spa, France, 1926.

6 — LA VIE AU MONT-DORE
Arrêtez ! Arrêtez ! J'ai le mal de mer !

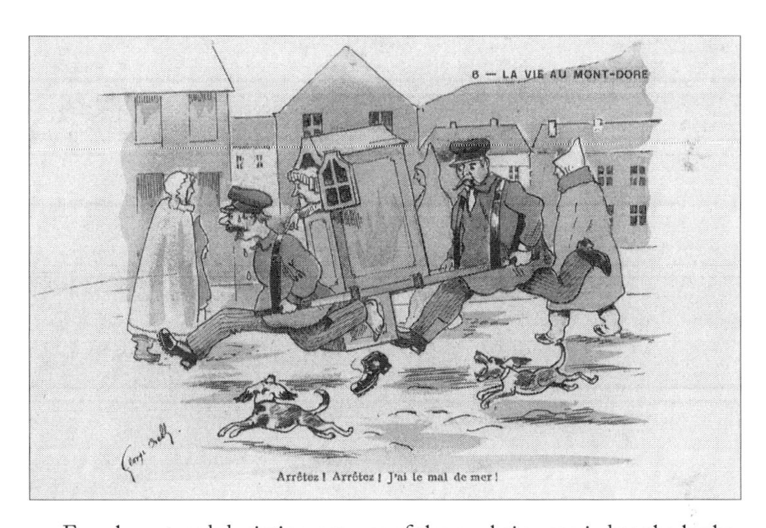

30 French postcard depicting patrons of the spa being carried to the baths.

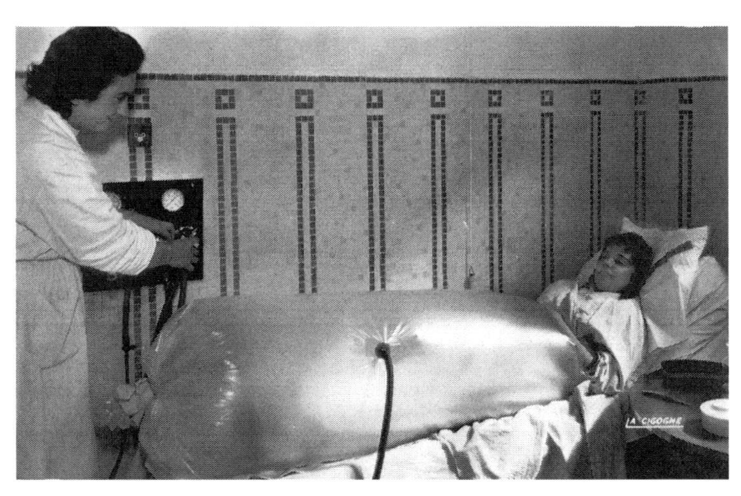

31 Early twentieth-century spa treatment with either steam or perhaps radioactive gas.

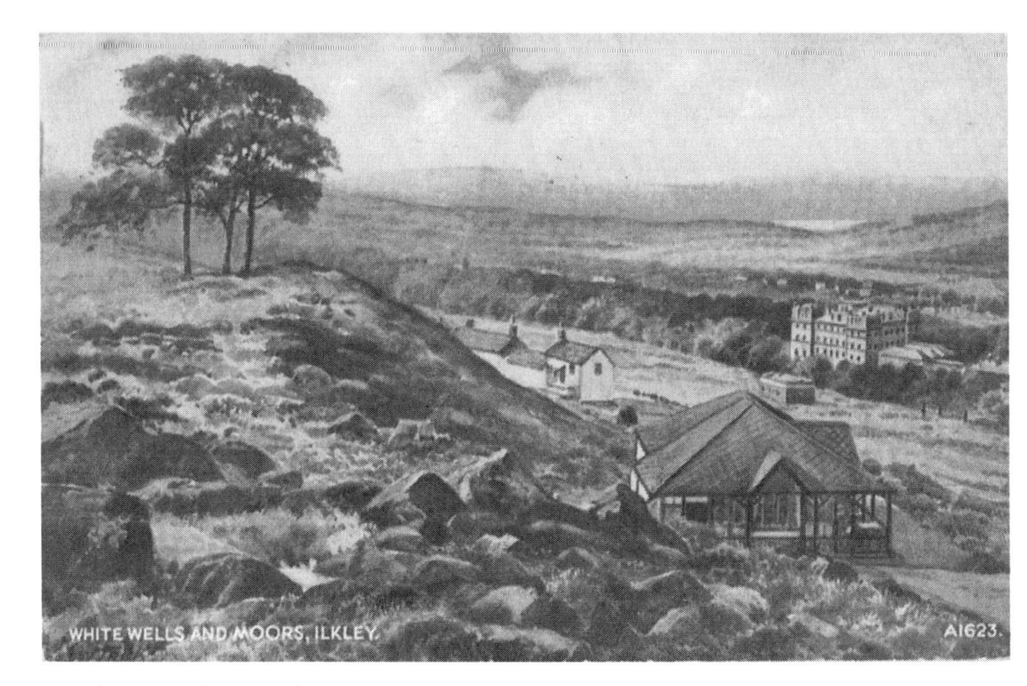

32 White Wells Spring and moors, Ilkley, Yorkshire.

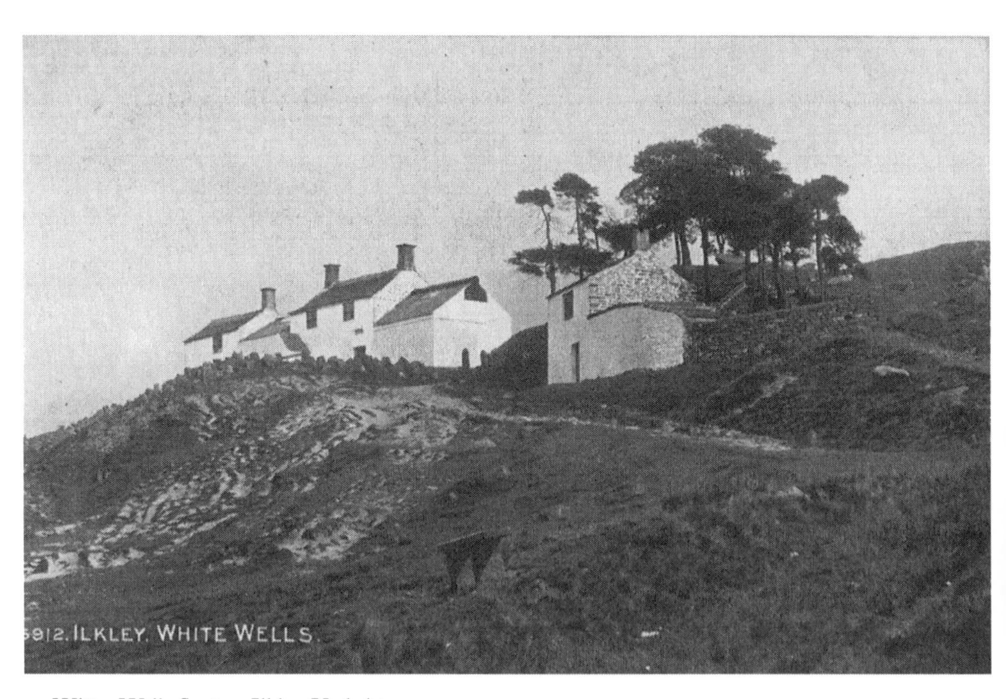

33 White Wells Spring, Ilkley, Yorkshire.

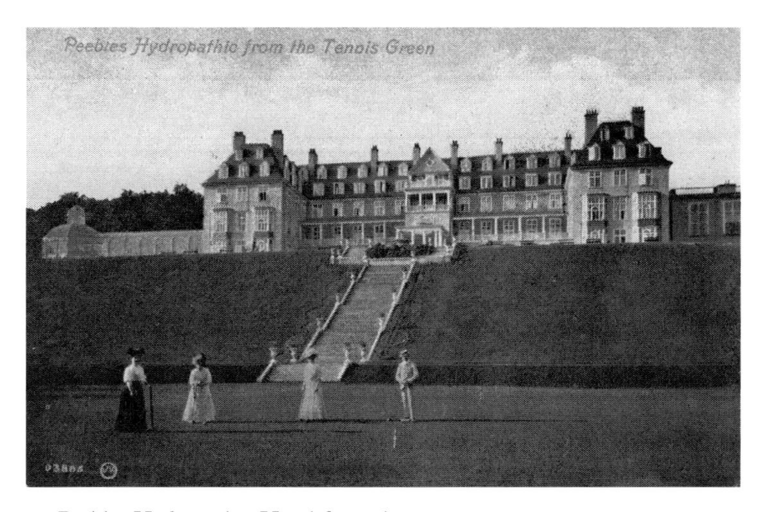

34 Peebles Hydropathic Hotel from the tennis green, 1917.

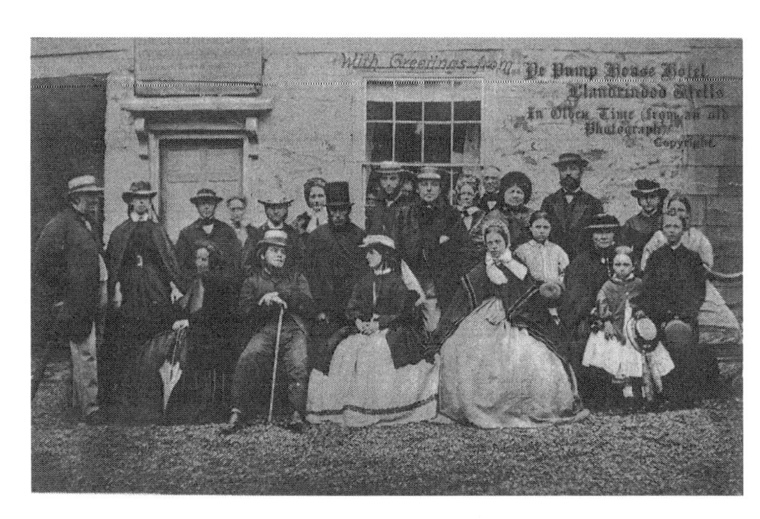

35 The Pump House Hotel, Llanrindod Wells, Wales.

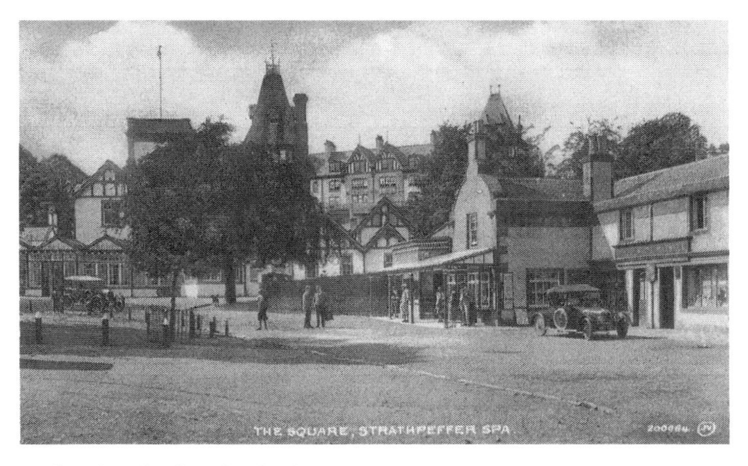

36 Strathpeffer Spa, Scotland, 1920s.

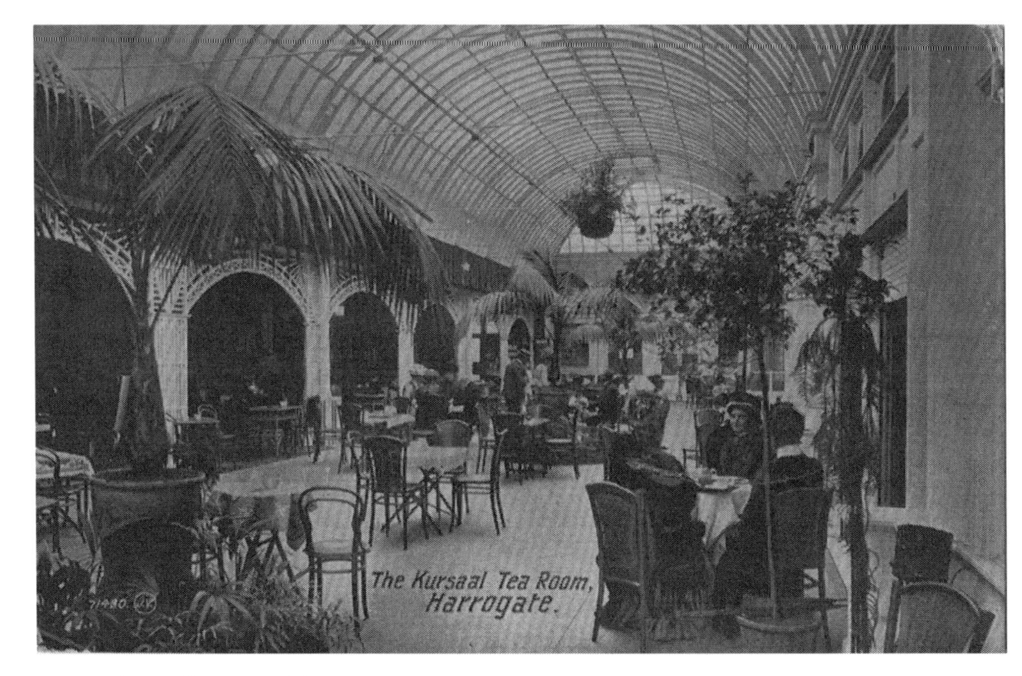

37 The Kursaal Tea Room, Harrogate, 1914.

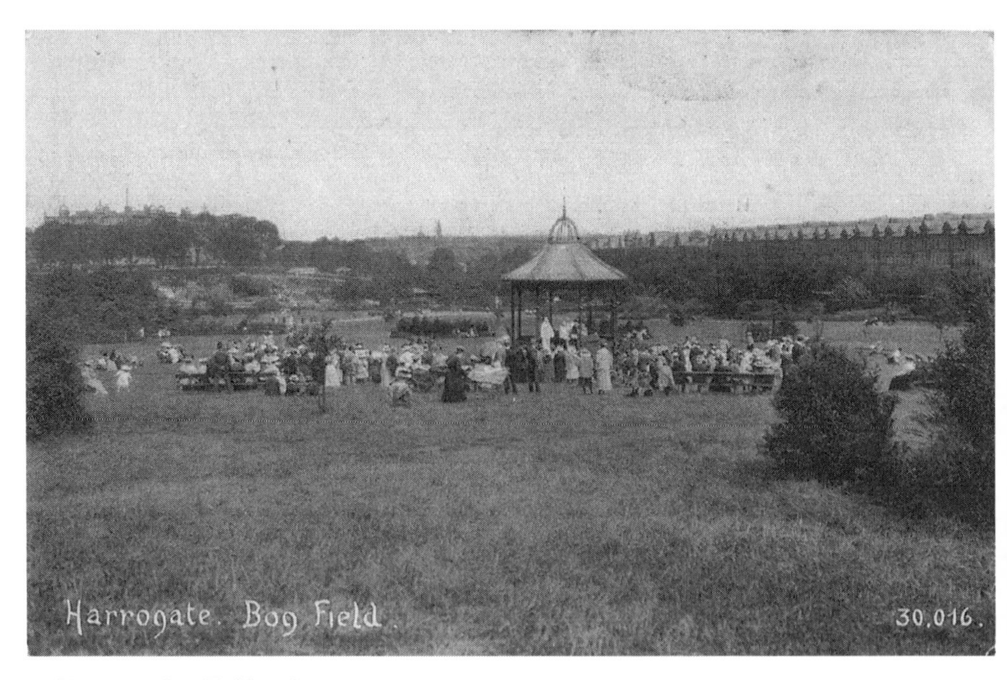

38 Harrogate, Bog Field, early 1900s.

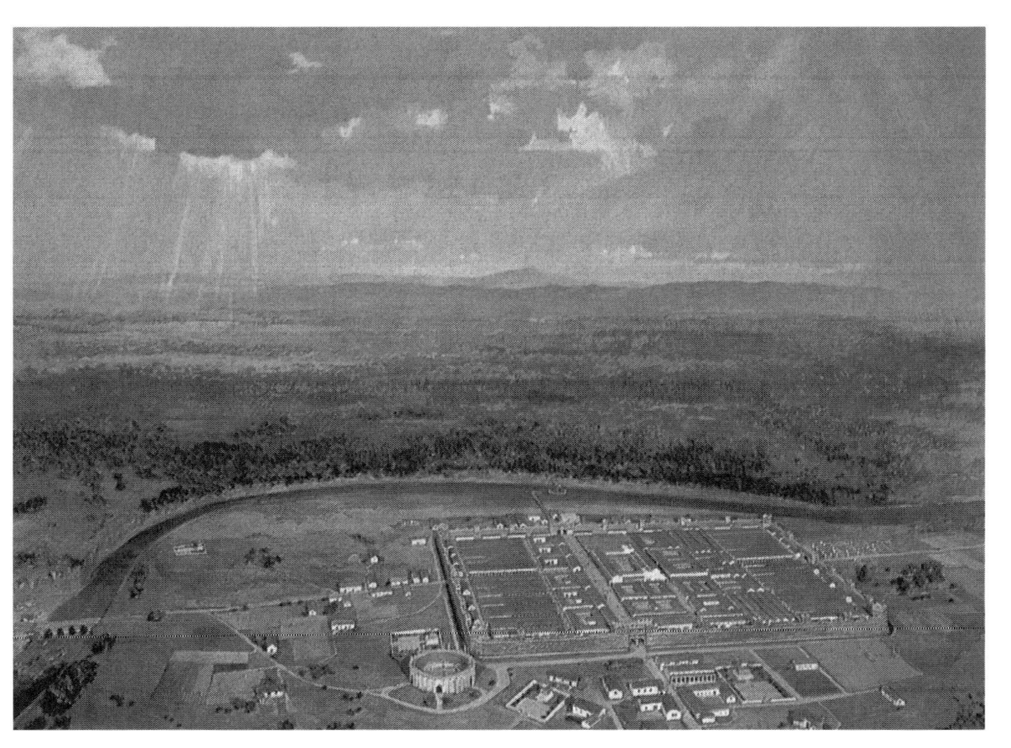

39 Reconstruction of the Roman legionary fortress at Chester and the crossing of the River Dee around AD 125.

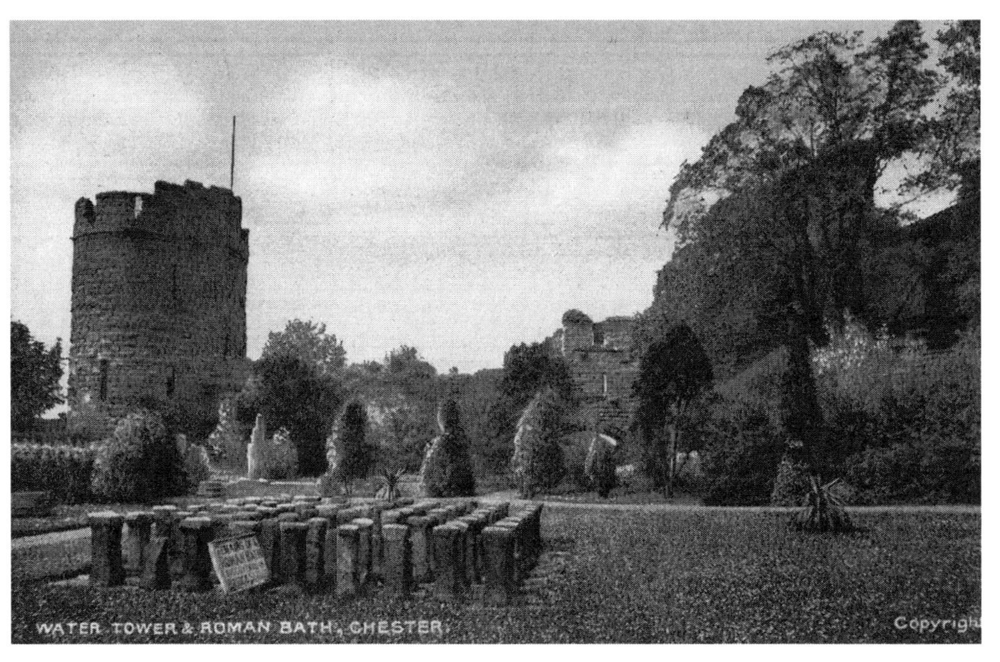

40 Water Tower and Roman Bath at Chester in Cheshire. Roman remains, part of the legionary baths, are located on Bridge Street in the basement of Spud-U-Like. The hypocaust in the Water Tower garden appear to have gone, perhaps relocated in the Roman Gardens.

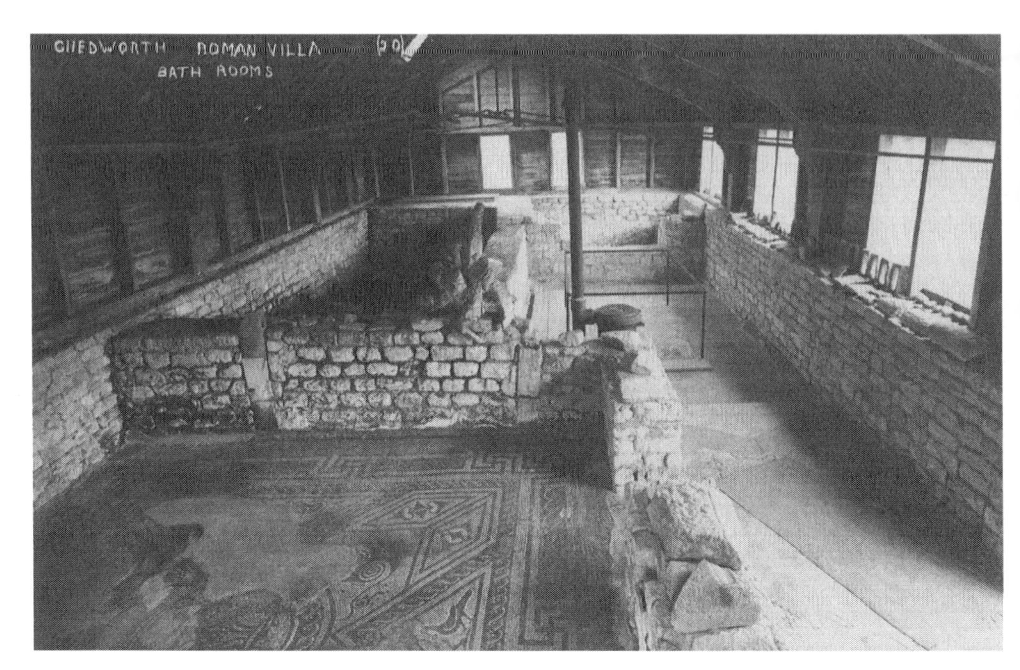

41 Chedworth Roman Villa, showing the bath rooms.

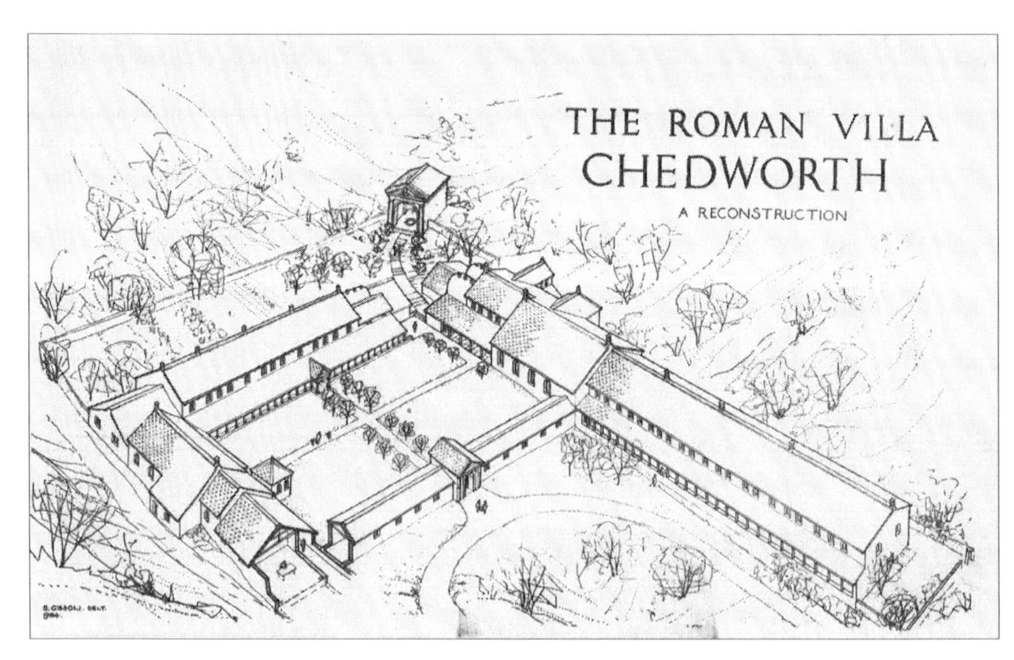

42 The Roman Villa, Chedworth.

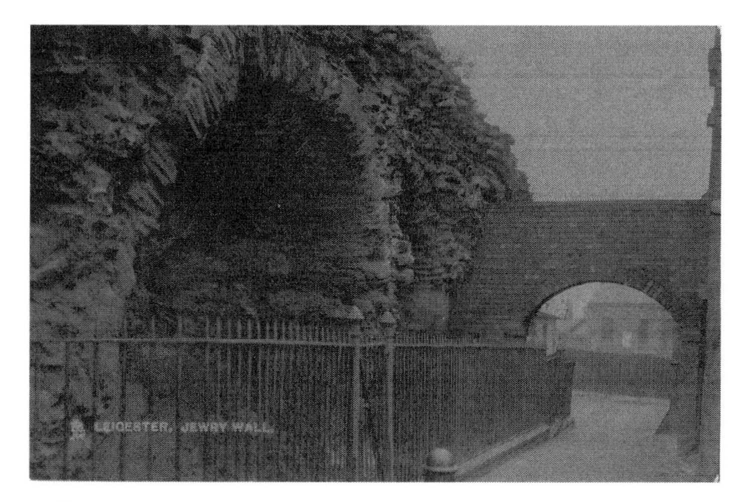

43 Jewry Wall, Leicester.

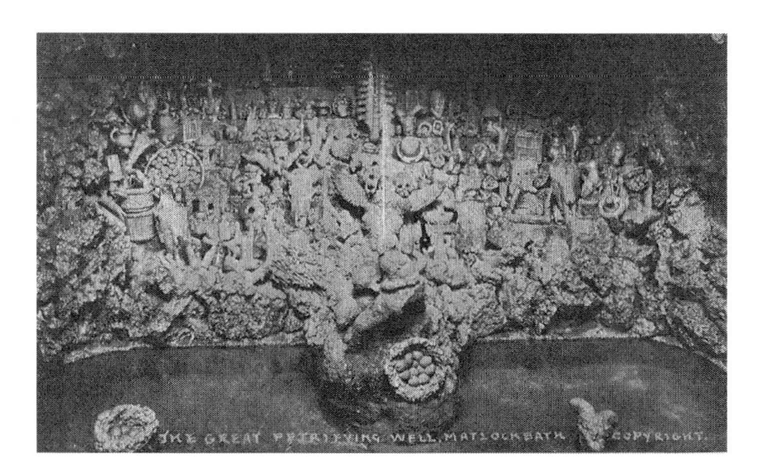

44 The Great Petrifying Well, Matlock Bath, 1920s.

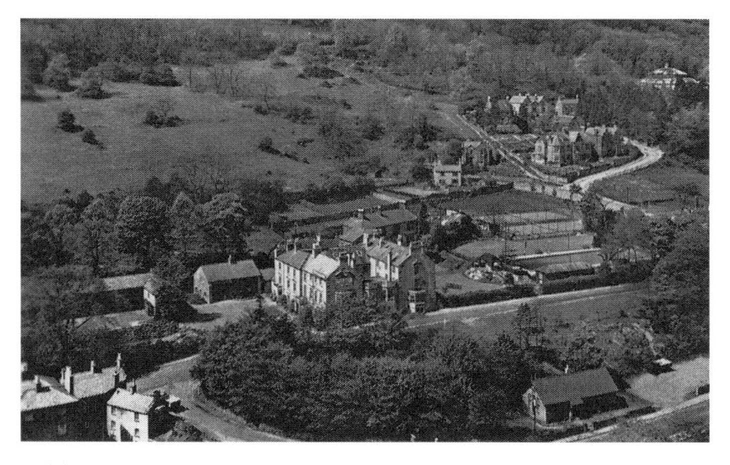

45 The New Bath Hotel, Matlock, 1951.

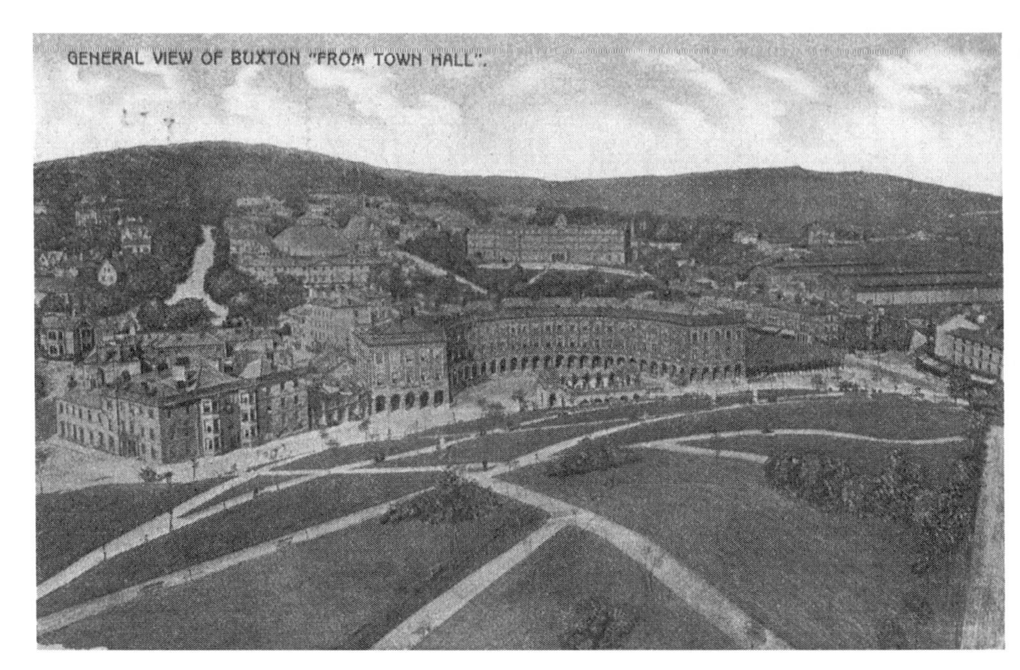

46 Buxton from the Town Hall, early 1900s.

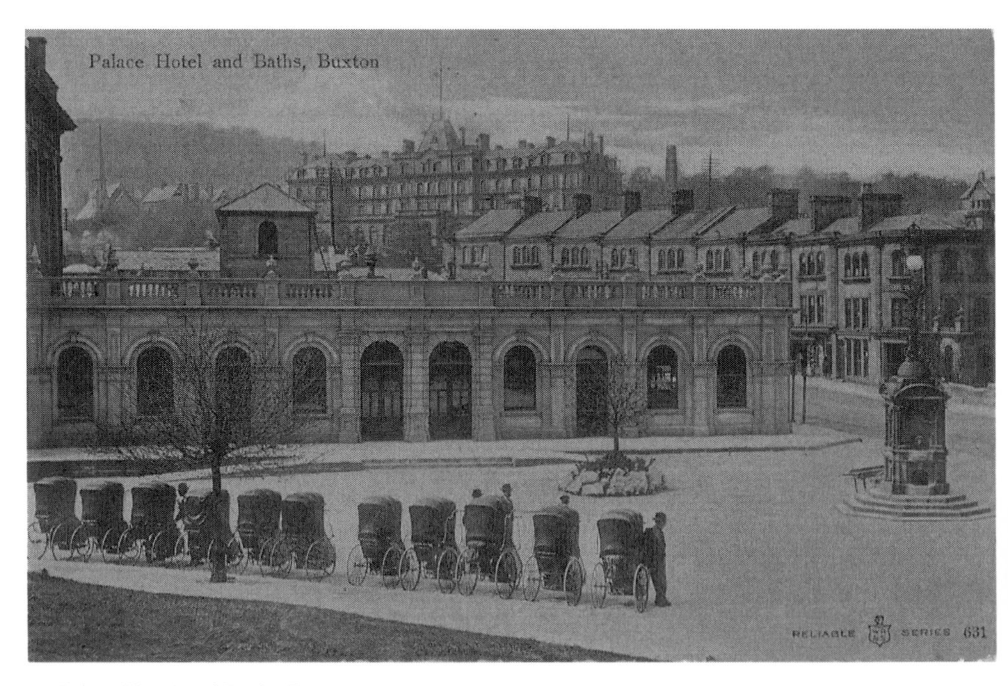

47 Palace Hotel and Baths, Buxton, 1905.

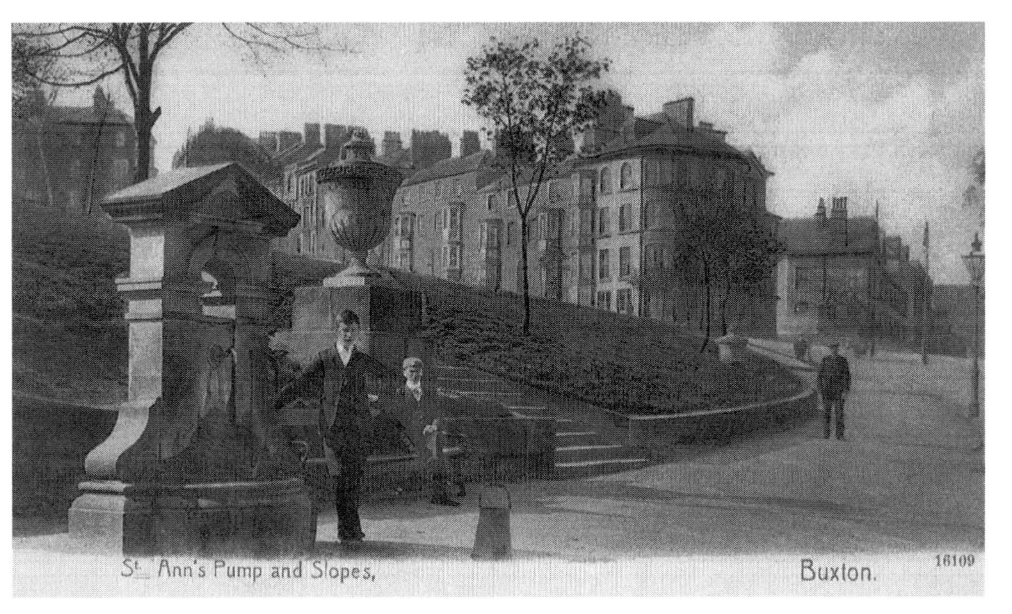

48 St Ann's Pump and Slopes, Buxton, 1905.

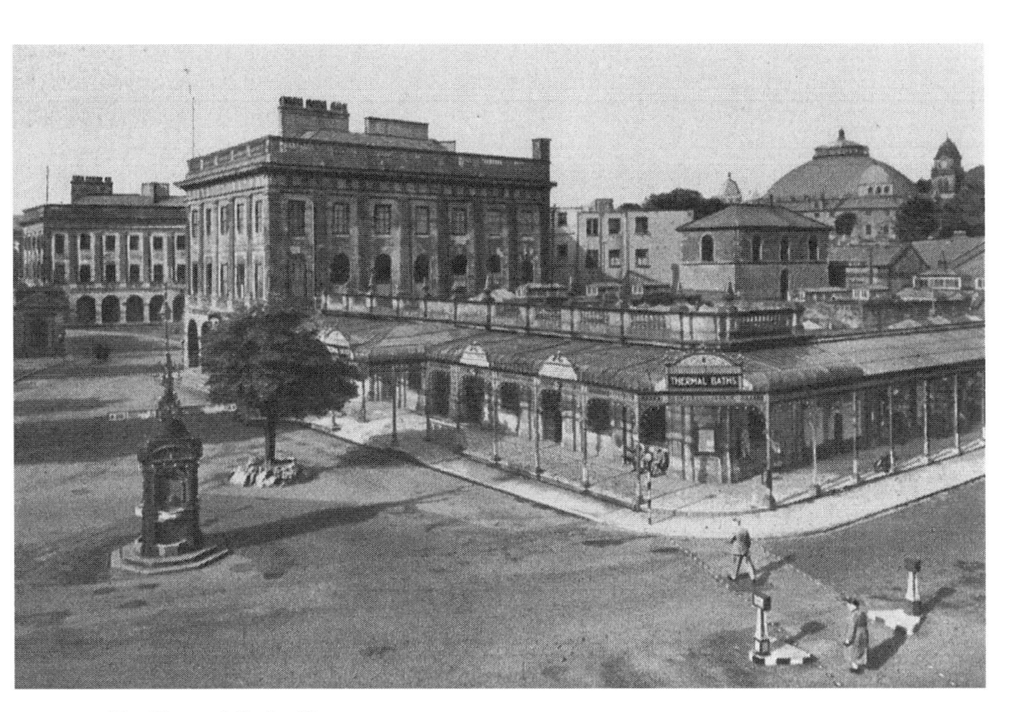

49 The Thermal Baths, Buxton, 1930s.

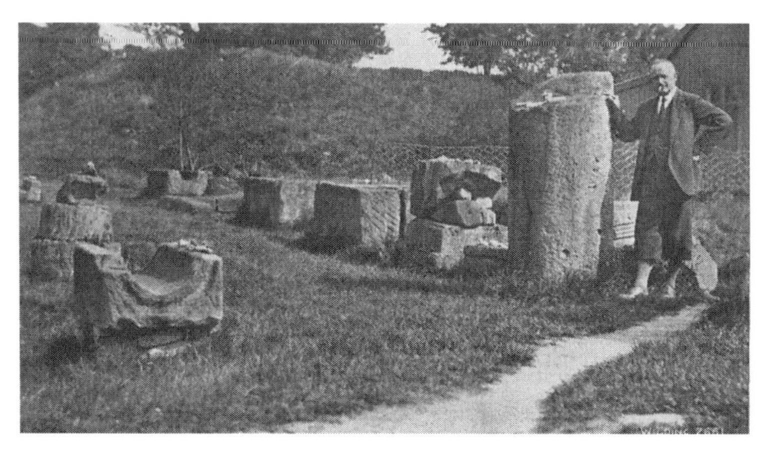

50 Passage from Watling Street leading to the Roman Bath, Viroconium.

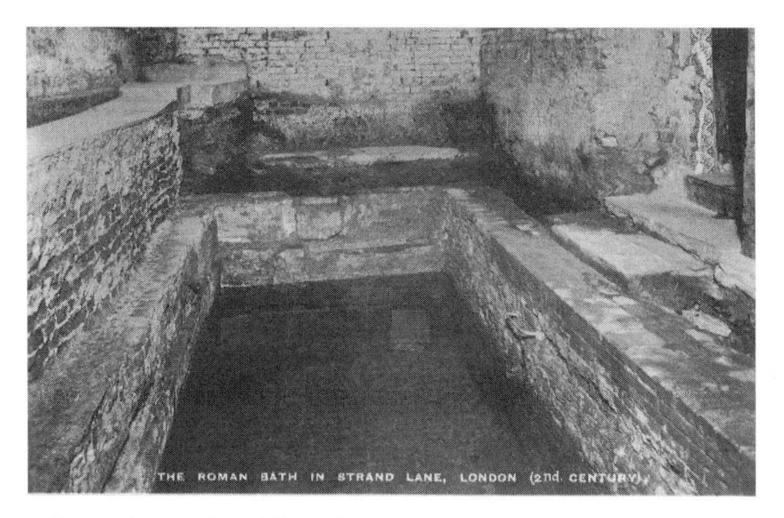

51 Roman Bath in Strand Lane, London, early 1900s.

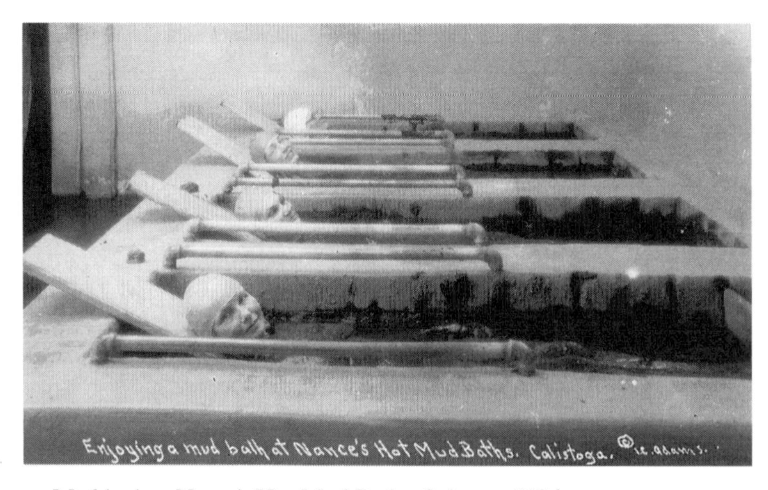

52 Mud bath at Nance's Hot Mud Baths, Calistoga, USA.

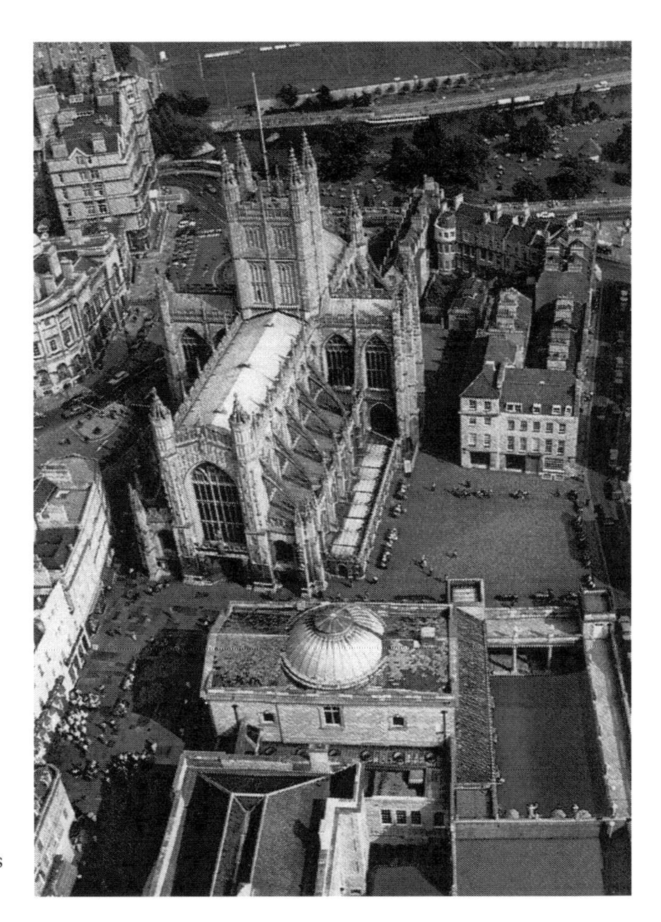

53 Bath Abbey and the Baths from the air.

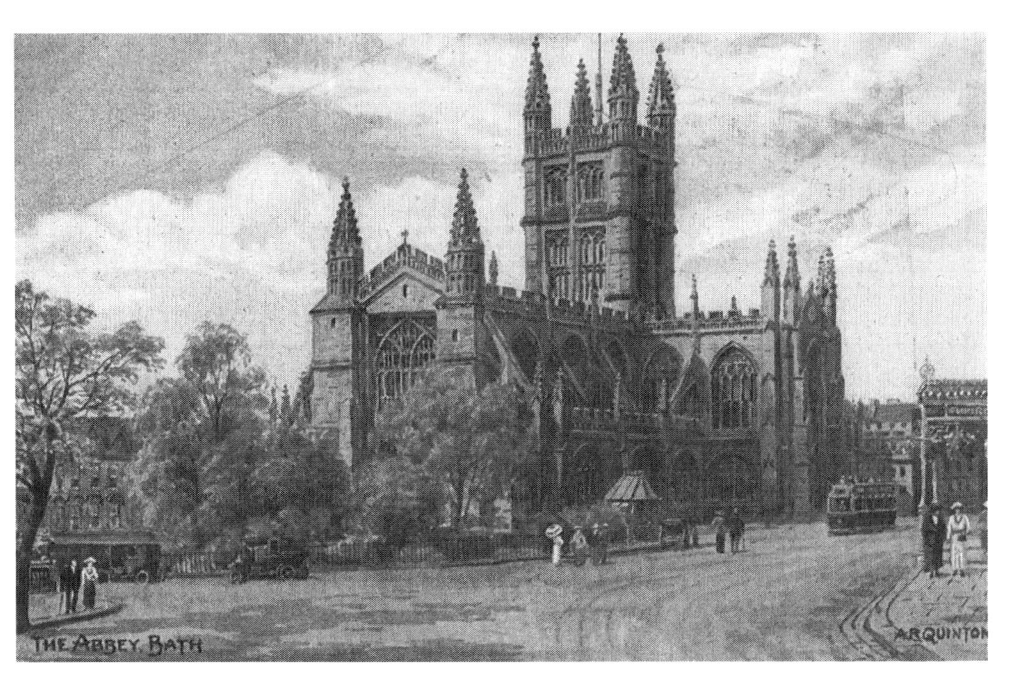

54 Bath Abbey, early 1900s.

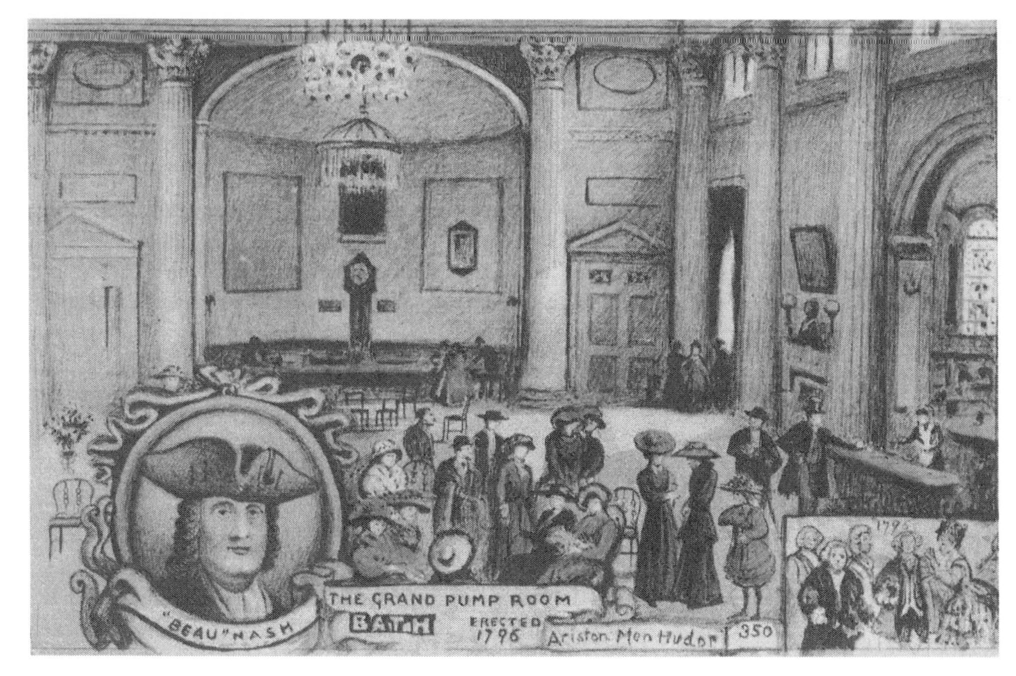

55 The Grand Pump Room, Bath.

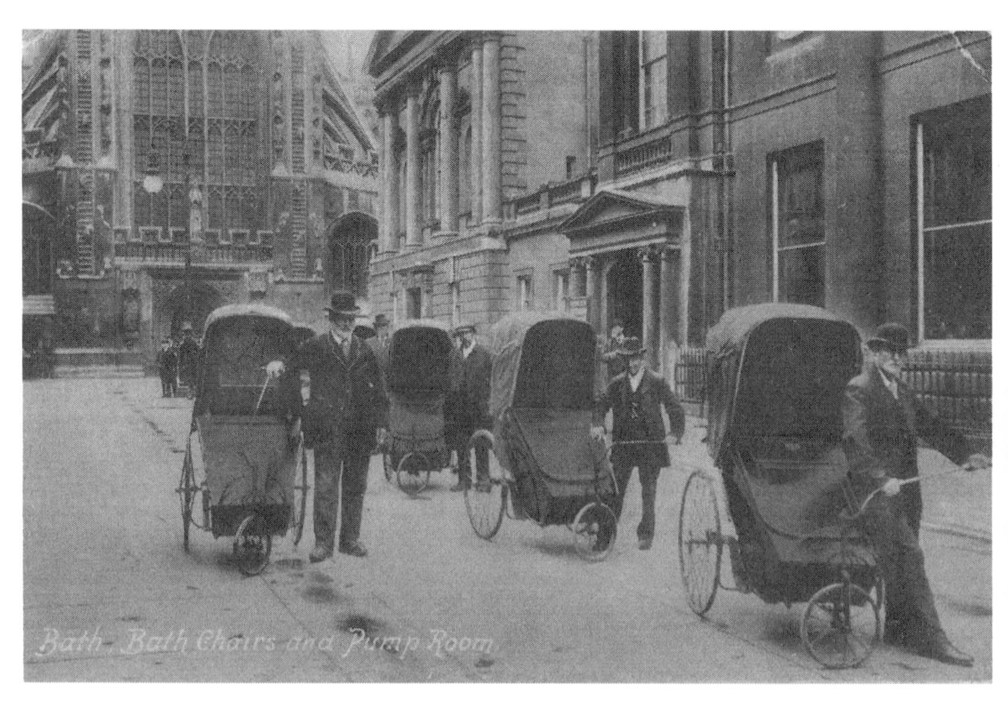

56 Bath Chairs and Pump Room, Bath.

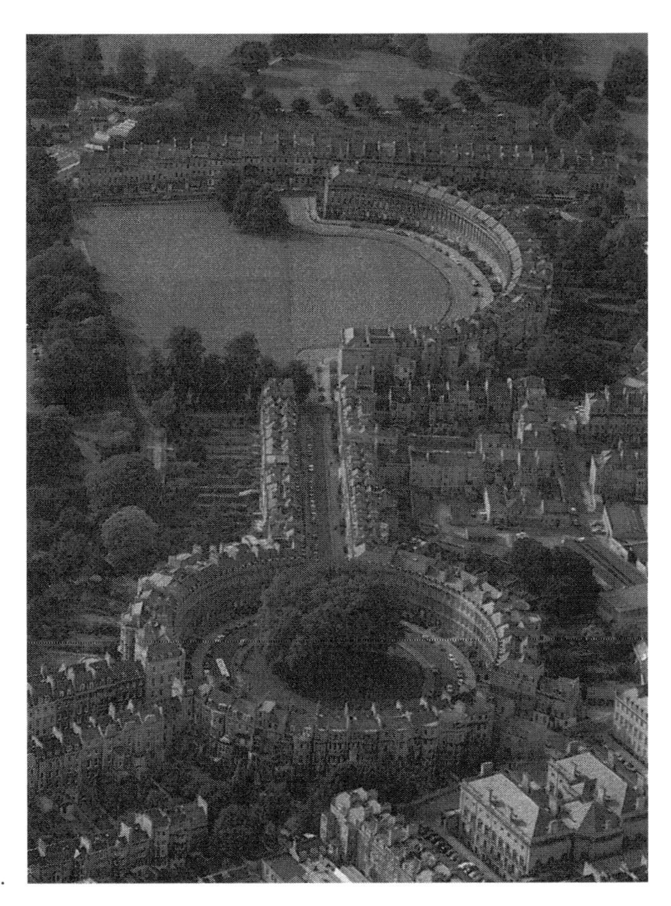

57 The Georgian City, Bath.

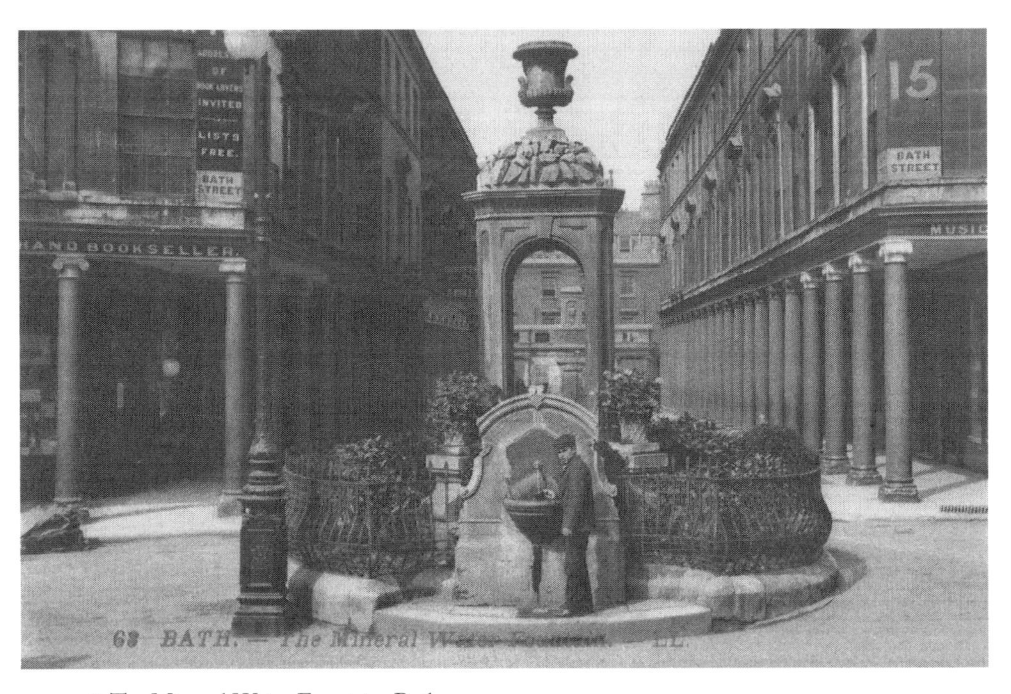

58 The Mineral Water Fountain, Bath.

Bath. The Roman Baths during first excavations. The Roman Baths were discovered in 1755, when the Priory was pulled down to make the Kingston Baths. Some of the old bricks were marked by fire, and soot was found still remaining from Roman days. Excavations were started in 1881.

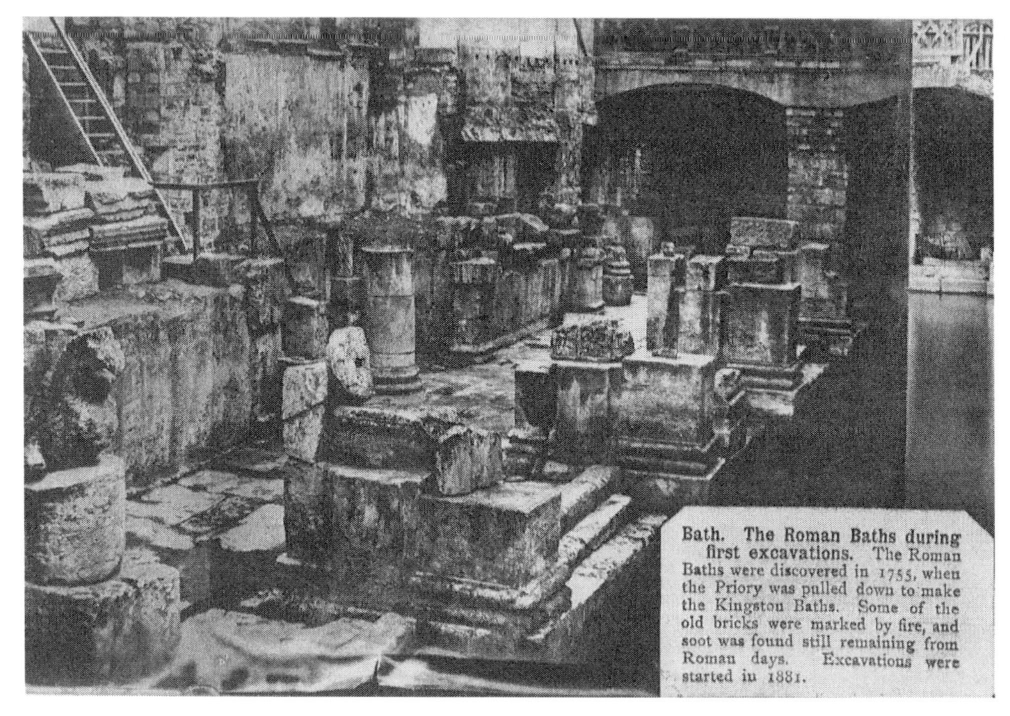

59 The Roman Baths at Bath during the first major excavations, which began in 1881.

25

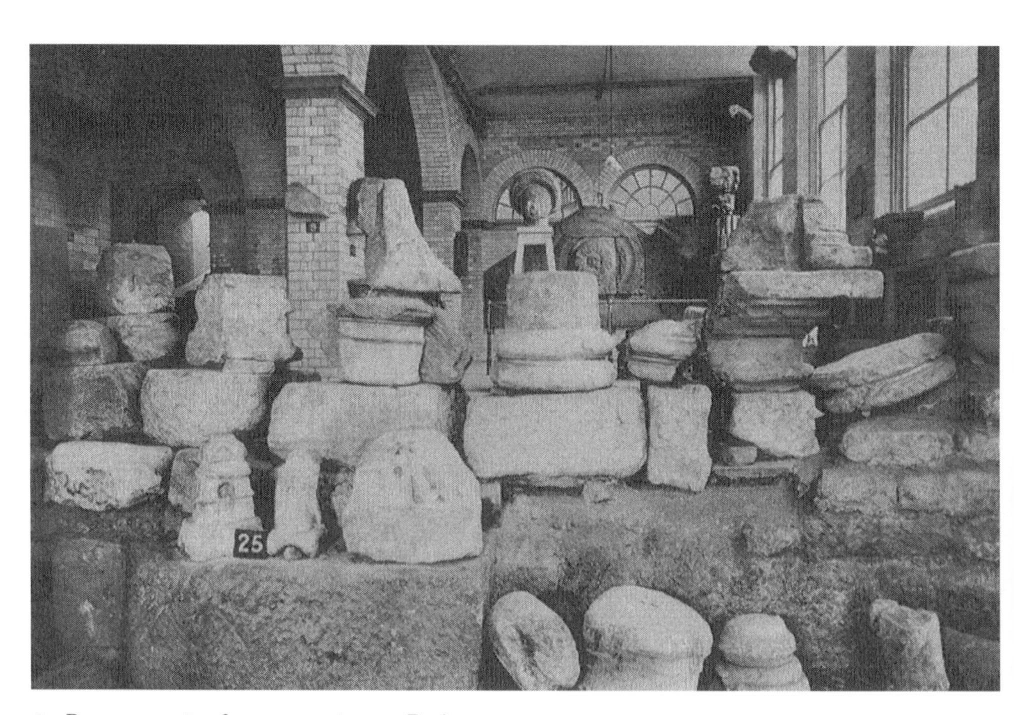

60 Roman remains from excavations at Bath.

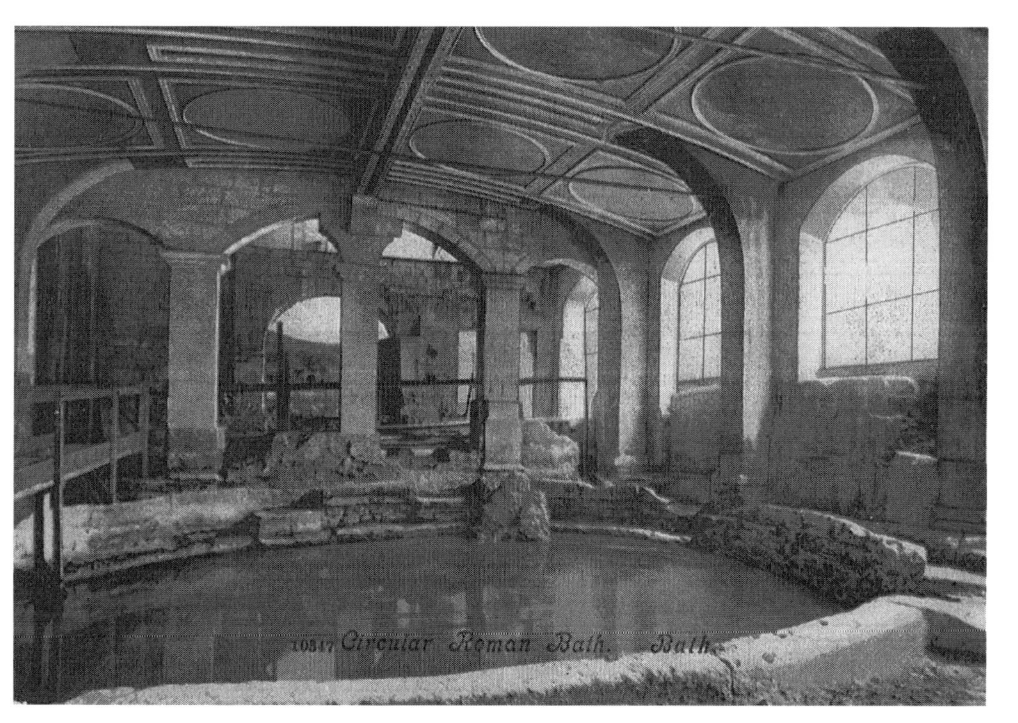

61 The Circular Roman Bath at Bath.

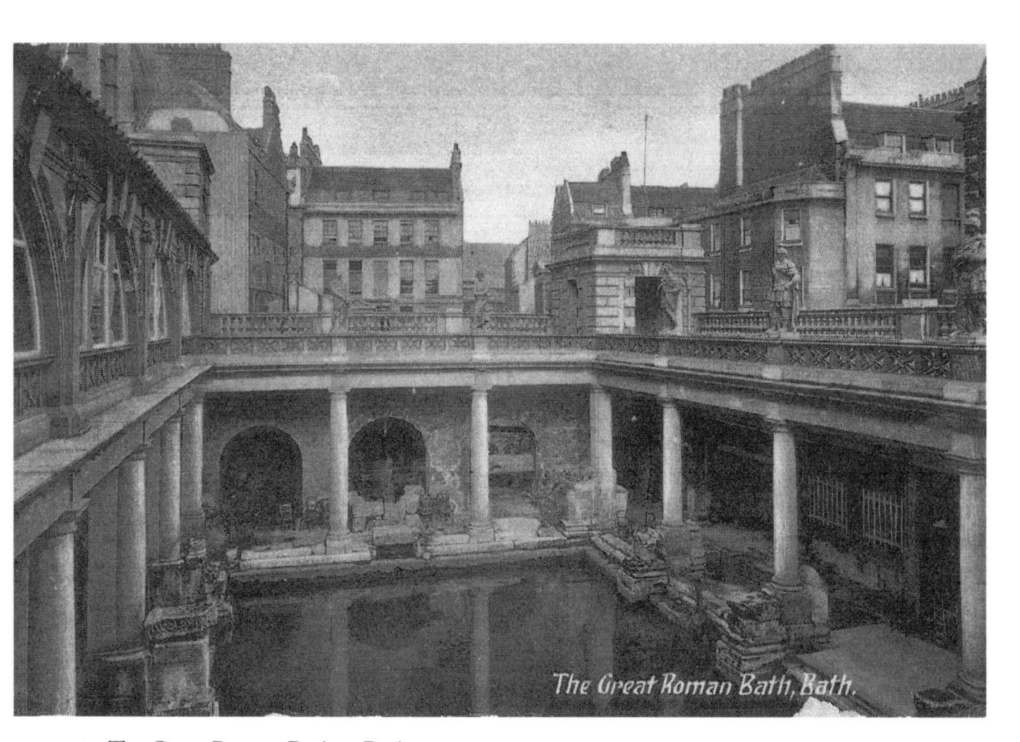

62 The Great Roman Bath at Bath.

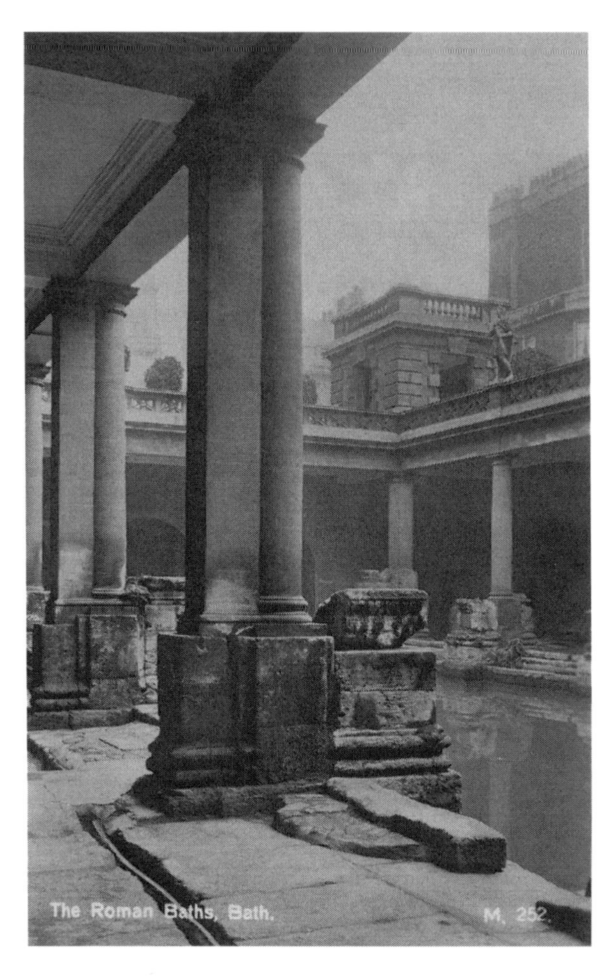

Left and below: 63, 64
The Roman Baths.

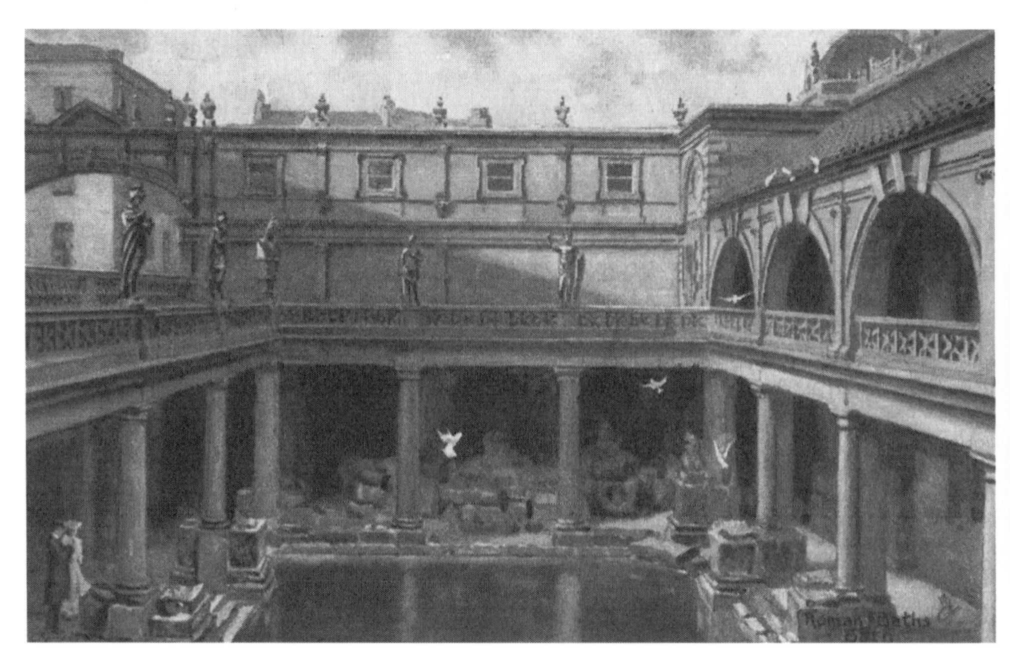

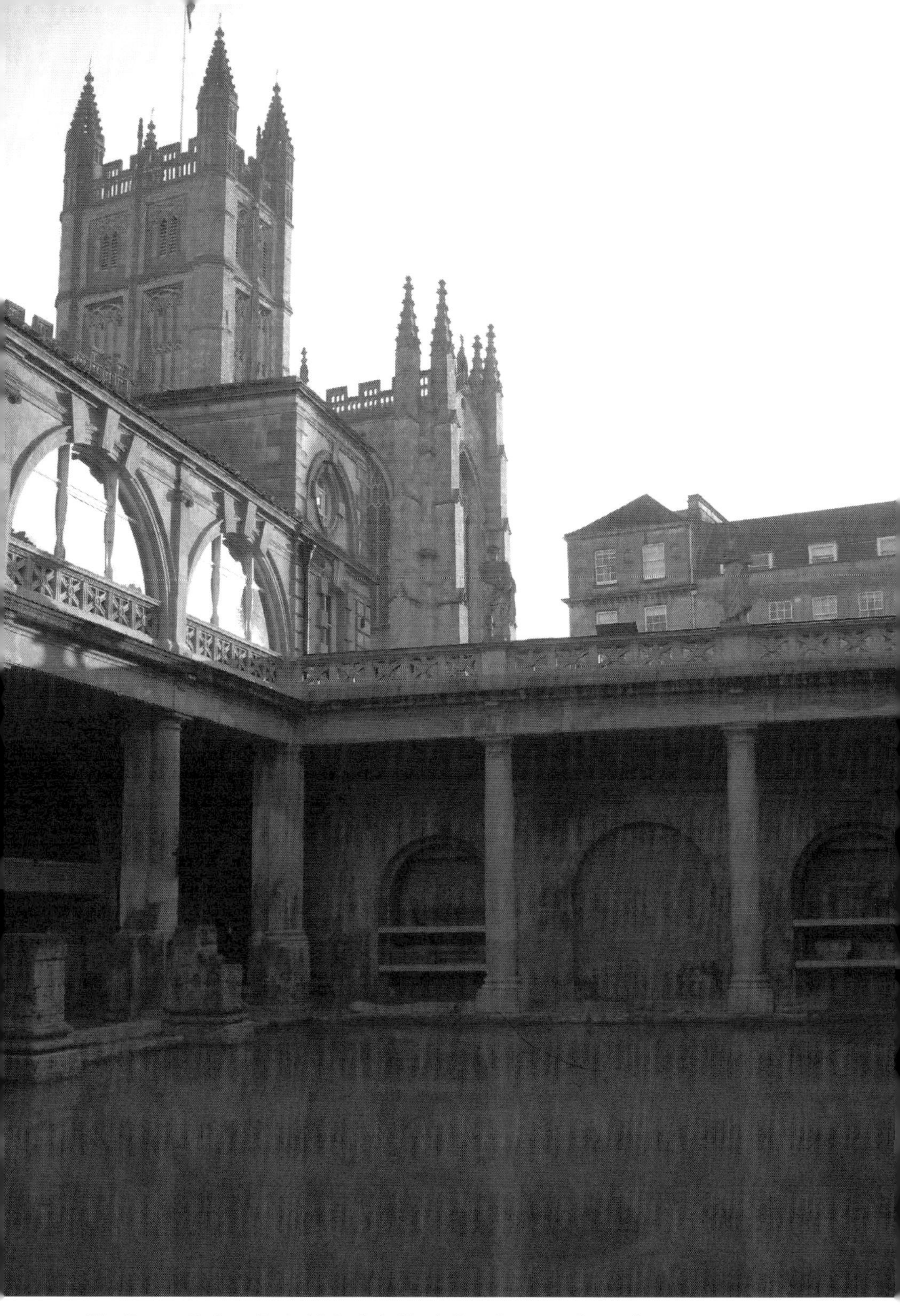

65 The Roman Baths at Bath. (© Bath & North East Somerset Council)

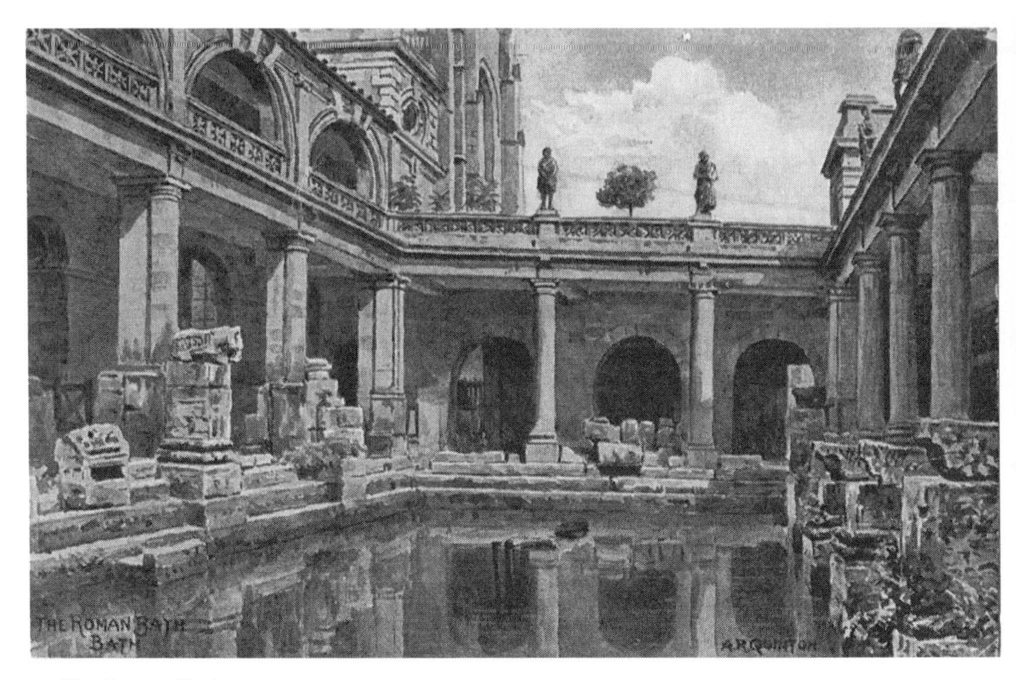

66 The Roman Baths.

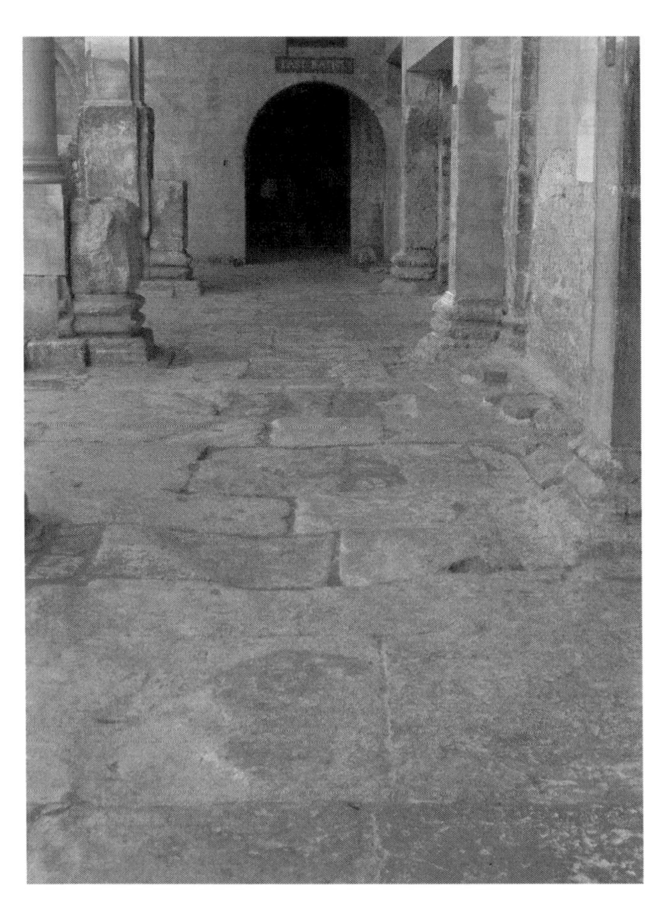

67 View towards the East Baths at Bath. (© Bath & North East Somerset Council)

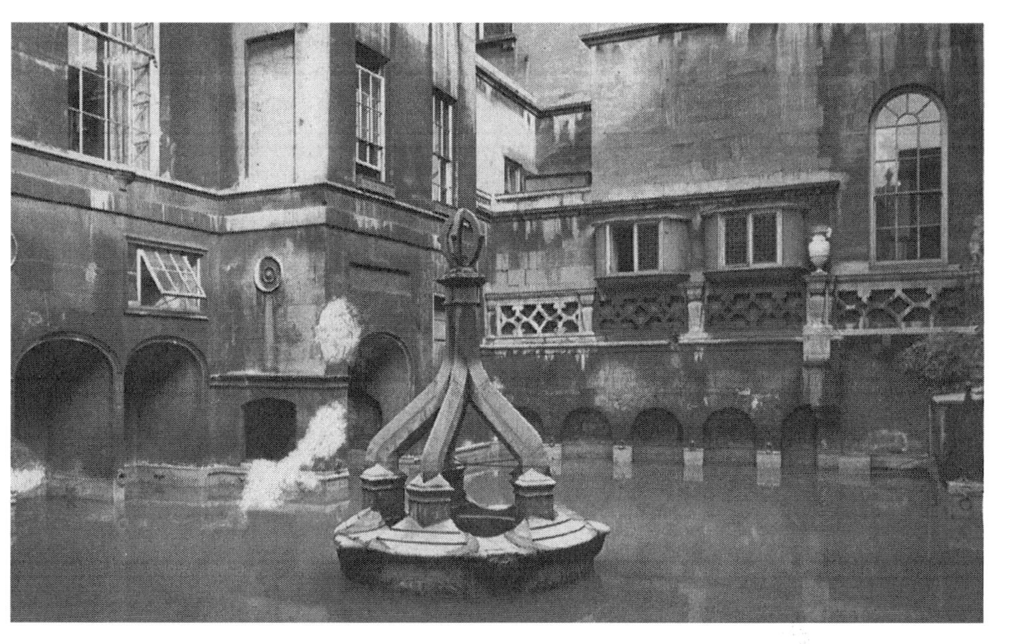

68 The King's Bath at Bath, 1952.

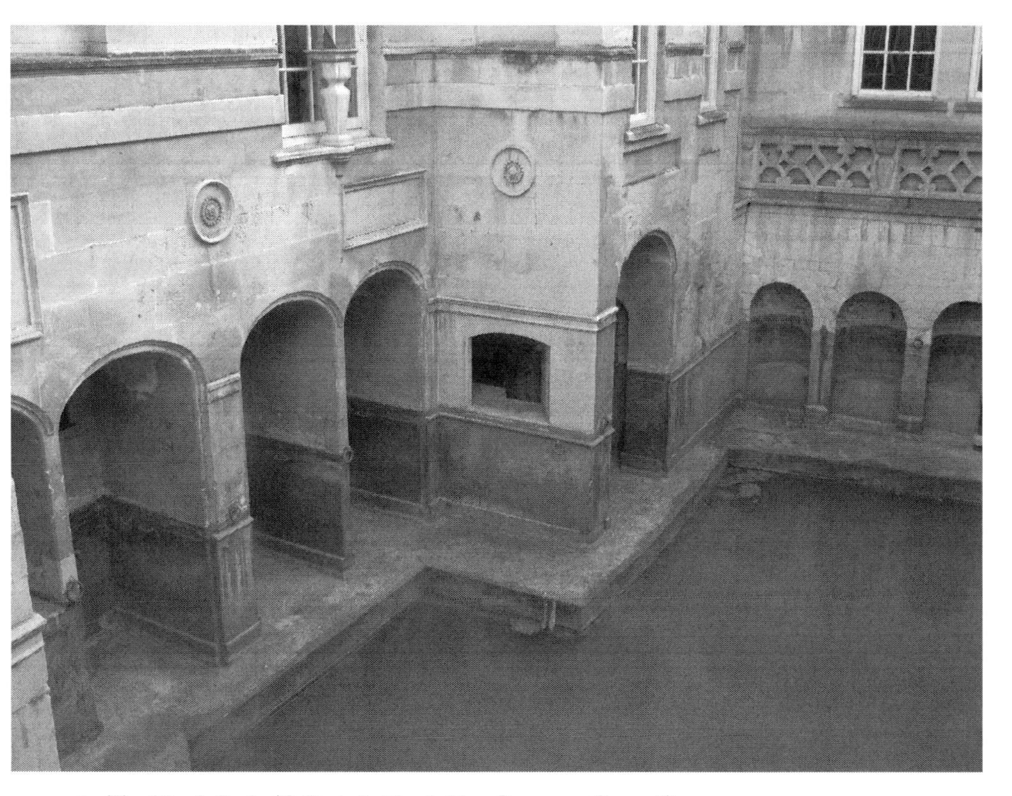

69 The King's Bath. (© Bath & North East Somerset Council)

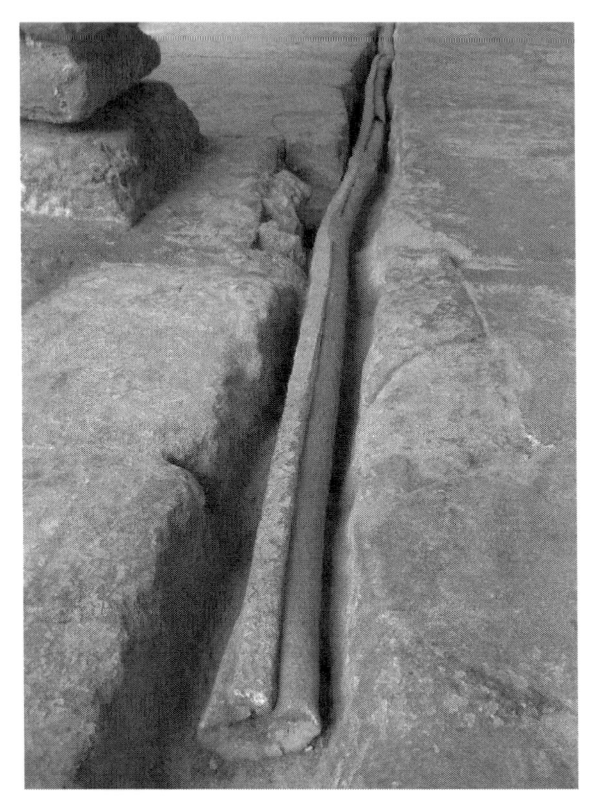

70 The lead pipe to supply water to the Great Bath at Bath. (© Bath & North East Somerset Council)

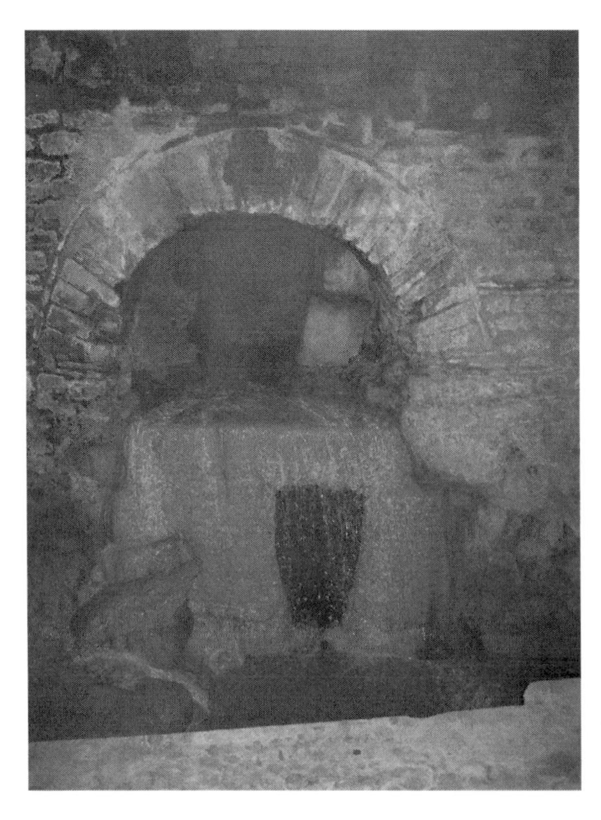

71 The Spring Overflow at the Roman Baths in Bath. (© Bath & North East Somerset Council)

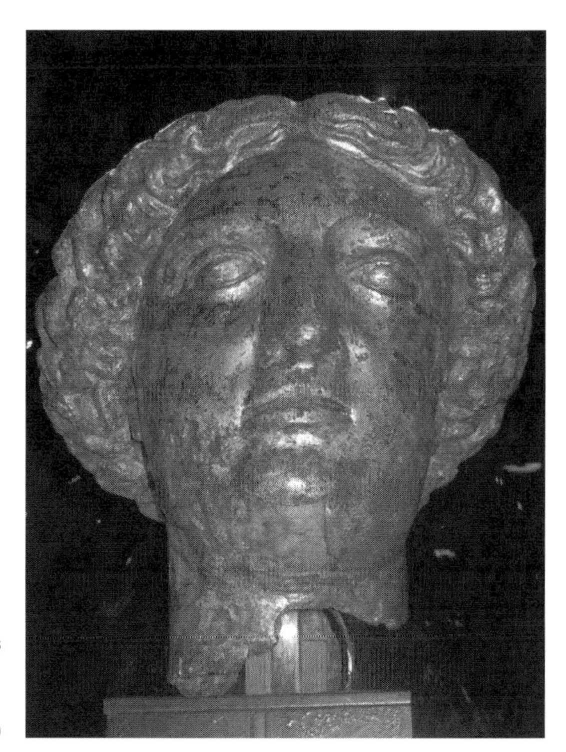

72 The gilt bronze head of the goddess Sulis Minerva on display at the Roman Baths Museum in Bath. (© Bath & North East Somerset Council)

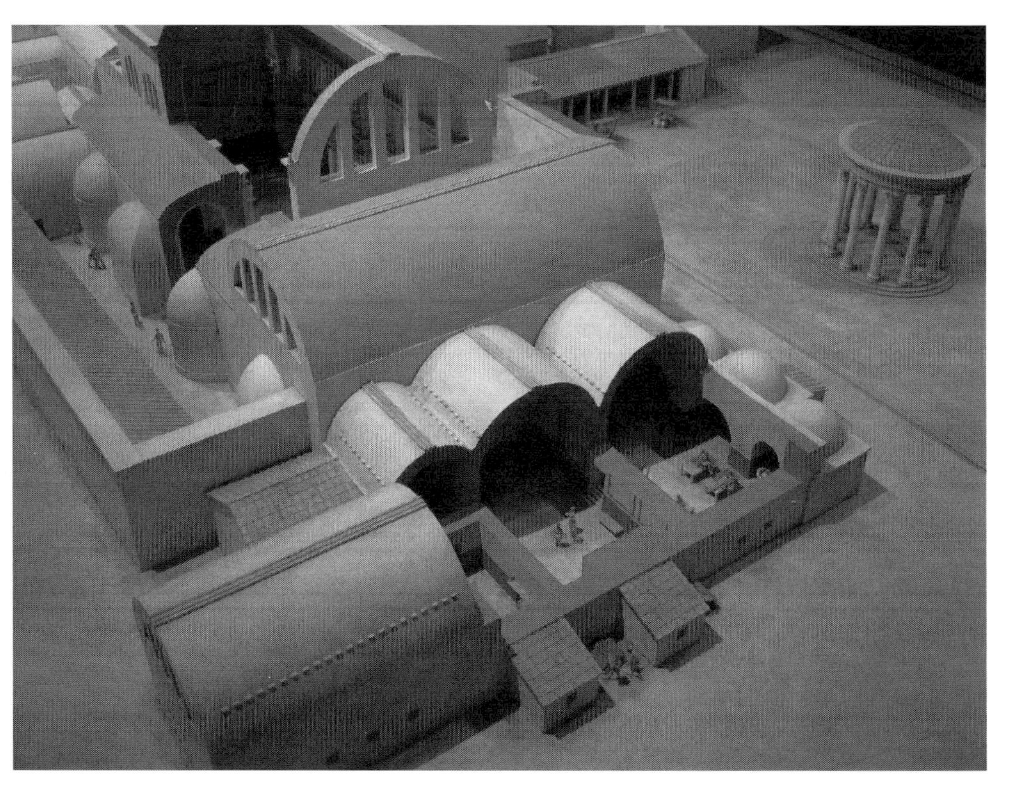

73 Model of the Roman Baths and temple complex at the Roman Baths Museum. (© Bath & North East Somerset Council)

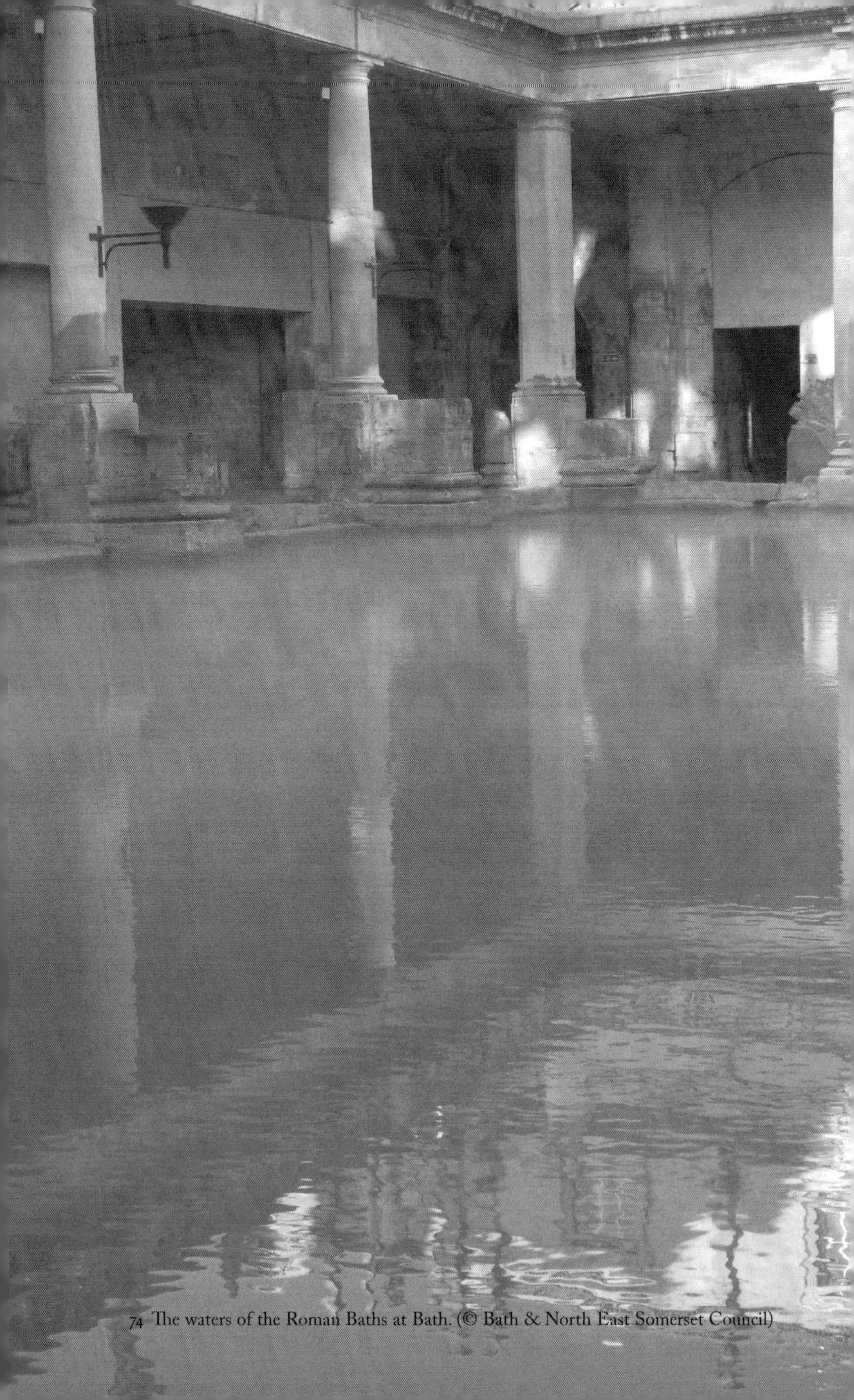

74 The waters of the Roman Baths at Bath. (© Bath & North East Somerset Council)

5

ROMAN BATHS IN GREAT BRITAIN

The Roman historian Tacitus described the Roman way of life with 'the lounge, the banquet, the bath', and asserted that this was 'a form of vice brought by the conquering Romans to Britain, which seduced the hardy native inhabitants of the island'. This chapter examines the places and sites that have known Roman baths and associated structures. It tells the stories of the most famous locations and explores what we have left today.

Tony Rook (1992 & 2002) provides a very useful gazetteer of the main sites of Roman baths in Britain. These sites were used as a starting point for the inventory below. However, in considering Roman baths and spas in Britain we need to consider that here is a complex heritage of wells, spas, and associated baths or bathhouses. Furthermore, this sits alongside a rich diversity of private baths attached to wealthy villas and farms, of military bathhouses, and the major public baths of the bigger towns and cities of the province. Of all these sites and remains there must be many for which the baths have never been discovered. Of the ones which are known to have existed, many have been swept away or at least been covered over by urban sprawl over the centuries. For those that are preserved, often all that is there are the structures left after nature and pillaging of bricks by later inhabitants of the same or nearby sites. Much of the above-ground structures have been 'robbed'.

So, at the end of all the decay of two thousand years, there is the heritage of some preserved buildings, a very limited continuity of bathhouse usage at health spas and maybe Bath itself. Then there is a mix of sometimes fanciful associations of sites, seventeenth- and eighteenth-century spas with earlier Roman use. The locations described below are the better known sites and many have monuments which can be visited.

Bar Hill, Strathclyde, Scotland: This is an open site at Twechar, approached by a footpath behind the war memorial. There are baths inside the Antonine Wall and they are of two periods. The extant features are outlines in turf but with some stone *pilae* still visible *in situ.*

Bath, Somerset, England: The baths are in the city centre near the abbey with splendid museums, bathhouses, and other tourist facilities. This is one of the most important Roman sites in southern Britain and is centred around a vast spa based on a uniquely hot spring. There are two main large suites of baths which have been subject to numerous changes and alterations over many centuries of history. The sites include the altar of the Temple of Sulis Minerva, with front steps exposed but underground. The old Roman sites include the Great Bath (about 25 metres by 12 metres) its floor covered with Mendip lead, the circular baths (perhaps used by women and children), the hypocaust and mosaic pavement and part of a Roman conduit. There have been many Roman finds associated with the area including in 1727, a bronze head of Sul Minerva, one of the finest Roman bronzes discovered in England. Following abandonment by the Romans the baths and other buildings were robbed of stone and bricks and were over-topped by sediments and the land and the drains were once again abandoned. Much of the above ground walls and structures around the baths as seen today have had phases of rebuilding and reconstruction but the lower levels, floor and foundations remain substantially from the Roman era.

It was as late as 1859 when the modern Pump Room was being built that a culvert was opened up to reveal Roman constructions. When this stonework was traced back to its source the 'Roman Baths', as they are known today, were exposed. Further investigation and excavation was done in the 1920s, and showed the extent of the eastern part of the bathhouse. Since that time, archaeological excavations were undertaken in the 1950s, 1960s, and then from the 1970s onwards, to give the picture of the Roman construction and the archaeological remains.

Bearsden, Strathclyde, Scotland: This is an open site located at 35 Roman Road around 140 metres north of the car park, with entrance through a small gate in the wall. Dating from around AD 65–142, the site has some interpretation. It is arguably the most impressive building along the Antonine Wall, with existing remains of a drainage system and latrine, and with stone *pilae* and jacketing.

Bignor, West Sussex, England: The site is located on a minor road running between Bury and Bignor, and is 8 km south-west of Pulborough. There is a museum on site and two suites of baths laid out with grass and gravel. The cold bath complex of one of the facilities is intact and excavation has shown considerable robbing of stone from other parts of the site.

Binchester, County Durham, England: The baths are situated on a minor road off the A689. They are located inside a minor fort called Vinovia, and are believed to have belonged to the commander. A new house with a luxurious bath-suite was built sometime around AD 350. The remains are under cover and today represent the best preserved hypocausted baths in Britain, including standing *pilae* which still support a concrete floor with flues still *in situ*. The site was discovered in the early nineteenth century but its archaeology was later badly damaged by treasure hunters.

Bothwellhaugh, Strathclyde, Scotland: This is an open site in Strathclyde Park west of the M74. There is on-site interpretation which explains how the baths, belonging to a small Roman fort, are close to the so-called 'Roman bridge'. They were in fact re-erected here following the flooding of their original site to form a water reservoir. They date from around AD 65–142.

Buxton, Derbyshire, England: As discussed elsewhere, Buxton was both an important English spa centre in the eighteenth century and later, and was a significant Roman settlement and thermal spa. Whilst Victorian antiquaries reported finding and seeing Roman bath remains, there is little to be seen today. The waters here are also 'thermal' but cooler than at Bath.

Caerleon, Gwent, Wales: This is a major site with an excellent museum and sophisticated interpretation. Parts of the stone-built, first-century legionary fortress baths are presented in a modern building constructed over the top of the site. There are also other earlier baths visible to the west of the huge amphitheatre. These baths pre-date the amphitheatre which was built around AD 80, and at that time they were modified to avoid obstructing one of the amphitheatre entrances. However, late, in about AD 125, they were finally demolished. Bathhouses were amongst the first buildings to be made from stone rather than wood and then, during the second century AD, more defences and buildings were constructed this way.

Caernarfon, Gwynedd, Wales: Segontium at Caernarfon was an auxiliary fort built by the Romans when they extended their influence far into Wales. The site dates back to AD 77. It was a remote outpost even in Britain, but is now a well-known Roman site, attracting thousands of visitors each year (although the museum is now closed until further notice). In this remote and warlike region, the fortress held a regiment of up to 1,000 auxiliary soldiers until about AD 394. These troops were non-citizens who were enrolled into army service for twenty-five years. This was a particularly strategic establishment, as it controlled access to Anglesey, the final homeland of the Druids. It also protected the Welsh coast from the sea-bound Irish raiders. Apart from its military functions, Segontium was the administrative centre for north-west Wales. The remains today include a major stone bathhouse constructed in the late third or early fourth century but seemingly never completed. The remains show typical cold, tepid and hot rooms, together with the furnace.

Chedworth, Gloucestershire, England: This National Trust property is found at the end of a minor road signposted from the A429 around 5 km north-west of Fossebridge. The complex includes two sets of baths situated in the corner of a most impressive courtyard villa. The smaller suite of baths has well-preserved flue-tiles and mosaics still *in situ*. The larger suite of baths is a complex, multi-period feature and part of an earlier bathhouse is outlined in turf.

Chesters, Northumberland, England: The baths are signposted from Chollerford on the B6318. These are the extramural baths of the Hadrian's Wall fort of *Cilurnum*, and as such are amongst the most famous upstanding Roman buildings in Britain. The harsh weather combined with stone robbing has caused damage to the remains, but nevertheless they are still impressive. The fort commandant's house has a small suite of baths and numerous heated rooms. The changing room has niches which may have been clothes lockers.

Colchester, Essex, England: Colchester was originally named *Camulodunum*, from the Romanisation of its Celtic name meaning the 'Fortress' (*-dunum*) of 'Camulos', the God of War. The earlier Iron-Age settlement was about 3 miles south-west of present-day Colchester. However, following the first-century Roman invasions Colchester was the site of the effective capital of the new colony and was a fine Roman town but, bizarrely, was largely undefended. Following the major East Anglian revolt, the town was burned to the ground, to be rebuilt when the rebellion was squashed. The conquering Romans this time moved their capital to the strategically placed Londinium. Today Colchester's Roman buildings are completely hidden by nearly two thousand years of subsequent occupation; though the shape of the Roman town is visible in the lines of the city walls and the main streets. Camulodunum became a *colonia* or planned town for military veterans who were given land within the settlement. This helped to establish and maintain a Roman presence in the subjugated territory. Essentially Colchester became Britain's first-ever city and as such – along with a significant military presence – it undoubtedly had baths, but they are not to be seen today.

Dorchester, Dorset, England: The baths are located in Colliton Park behind the County Hall, and the southern group of Romano-British buildings, from AD 300–400, have been suggested to be a suite of baths.

Droitwich, Worcestershire, England: The town of Droitwich Spa, the name of which is often abbreviated to just Droitwich, is located in north Worcestershire on the banks of the River Salwarpe. The reason for the town's significance as a spa is that it is situated on massive deposits of salt and these have been exploited since ancient times. The natural brine found at Droitwich contains 2½ lbs (about 1 kg) of salt per gallon, ten times stronger than sea water. Indeed, it is said to be rivalled only by the waters of the Dead Sea. In Roman times the village where Droitwich now stands was known as Salinae and was located at the crossroads of several Roman roads. Excavations have revealed Roman mosaic remains and a Roman villa or corridor-house around 40 metres long. Although Droitwich became a major spa town in the eighteenth century, it is not known to what extent it was a watering place in Roman times. However, even before Roman occupation it was a major centre for salt production and for the Romans was an important location for the industrial manufacture of salt. It seems likely that there would have at least been a major bathhouse to service all the people working and conducting business in the area.

In the mid-nineteenth century, Droitwich became famous as a spa town. Unlike other places, the medicinal benefits were not derived from drinking the spa water, which in this case is concentrated brine. At Droitwich the visitors swam and floated in the dense, concentrated salt solution and this gave muscular relief. The original use followed the outbreak of cholera in 1832, during which the wealthy patrons of local physicians were advised to take frequent hot baths. The salt-workers, not having such opportunities simply leapt into the warm brine barrels an his apparently had the desired effect. Indeed, the wealthier citizens we so impressed by the apparent health benefits to the workers that they d began taking hot brine baths, and a very lucrative enterprise was born. The town's brine baths, which first opened in the 1830s, were supplied by spa water which is some of the warmest in the United Kingdom outside Bath. It is not really a 'hot' spring since the ambient temperature of the water is below human body temperature. The Baths here were renowned for the treatment of rheumatic disorders. The original Brine Baths closed long ago, but a new brine bath opened to the public for relaxation and hydrotherapy as a part of the Droitwich Spa private hospital, but closed for financial reasons in December 2008.

The importance of Droitwich to the Romans and indeed to later people cannot be overemphasised. In a world without rapid transport and refrigeration, salting food to preserve it was incredibly important and the salt was a very valuable product, not just a condiment.

Ebchester, County Durham, England: Here the baths are in the gardens of Mains Farm, and the site is located opposite the church to the south of the A689. The ruins are from an internal suite of baths from the Roman fort of Vindomora, and the channel hypocaust of a single apsidal room is visible on site.

Exeter, Devon, England: The fort at Exeter was founded in the mid-50s AD as a small military fortress covering around 20 hectares. However, the location boasts a large stone-built bathhouse with one of the biggest sets of heated rooms in Roman Britain.

Fishbourne, West Sussex, England: The remains are to be found off Salthill Road, approximately 2.4 km from the A27 at Chichester. There is a museum and interpretation such as guidebooks. The overall complex is described as a palace and includes the remains of a small suite of baths that were built in around AD 100 and demolished some time about AD 270. The remains have been reconstructed and set in concrete and so features such as *pilae* are not in their original locations.

Hardknott, Cumbria, England: The baths here are located in the spectacular scenery of the Lake District's Hardknott Pass. The bathhouses here are external to the fort of Mediobogdum and are situated about halfway down the western pass. Relatively recent stone-robbing has led to the loss of a tile stoke-hole and hypocaust *pilae*, but a good circular *laconium* remains. In the remote Cumbrian Mountains, the fort was in use from late in the first century AD to the early second century. Afterwards, it was used as a roadside resting place for travellers.

Housesteads Roman Fort, Northumberland, England: This well-known site is located on Hadrian's Wall about 3 km north-east of Bardon Mill (off the B6318). The remains include two suites of baths with one adjacent to the commandant's house, and the other constructed into the barrack block close to the main gate.

Ilkley, Yorkshire, England: In the seventeenth and eighteenth centuries the town became fashionable for the curative benefits of its waters. Then in the nineteenth century Ilkley became a popular spa town and destination with the construction, between 1843 and 1844, of the Ben Rhydding Hydro, a Hydropathic Establishment at Wheatley about a mile away. Tourists flocked to 'take the waters' and bathe in the cold water spring. Wheatley was renamed Ben Rhydding after the Hydro, which has since been demolished. Development of the town followed the Hydro movement of the 1800s, and the associated establishment of a number of convalescent homes and hospitals. Good railway connections helped to encourage people to flock to the town's healing waters. Notable Victorian visitors included Madame Tussaud and Charles Darwin. The latter had hydropathic treatment at Wells House as his book *On the Origin of Species* was being published in November 1859. He and his family stayed at North View House (now Hillside Court). The only remaining Hydro building is a white cottage known as 'White Wells House', close to the moorland edge above the town itself. It is this site which has claims to a Roman association. The suggestion of a strong watering place and bath link for Ilkley in Roman times has been strengthened by the discovery of an altar stone dedicated to the Romano-British water goddess Verbia. This is inscribed:

> *Verbiae Sacrum Clodius Fronto D Praef. Coh II Lingon* or To sacred Verbia. Clodus Fronto, Prefect of Cohort, Second Legion.

However, the modern development is far more recent. In the 1700s, Ilkley's growth as a spa town began at White Wells on the town's outskirts and almost halfway to Ilkley Moor itself. The white-washed building was then just a two-room cottage. According to local history, sometime around 1780, a shepherd had an accident and severely damaged his leg. At first the wound wouldn't heal, but by with washing in the healing 'waters of Ilkley', the injury got better. The reputation spread and White Wells began to receive visitors seeking for themselves the therapeutic waters. Quite when the Roman claim developed seems shrouded in mystery. As a major Roman garrison town, Ilkley certainly had a Roman bathhouse. The White Wells seems an unlikely candidate for the site of the baths though the pure, cold water spring behind the Wells would be known to the Romans and perhaps have some significance.

The town has significant Roman associations with the remains of a Roman fort on a site near the town centre on the southern side of the River Wharfe. This may be Olicana, dating from AD 79 and it is suggested that from this was derived the name 'Ilkley'. But there is some disagreement. The site is now an Elizabethan manor house converted to a museum and there are a number of Roman altars from the reigns of Antoninus Pius (AD 138–61), and Septimius Severus and his son Caracalla (AD 211–17). The Romans arrived here around AD 79, and sections of the original Roman wall are visible in the gardens of the manor house. More evidence of Roman fort is to be seen close to All Saints Church.

King's Weston, Bristol, England: The Baths are part of a late third-century Romano-British villa located 3 km north of Sea Mills.

Lancaster, Lancashire, England: Lancaster has long been an important strategic settlement and its Roman baths are situated below the Priory. They are found about 100 metres from the path by the Wery Wall and the original structure was cut through by the fortifications built around the fourth century AD.

Leicester, Leicestershire, England: The Roman Baths at Leicester are one of the city's great surprises for visitors. They are located in the city centre with a museum and are close to modern university buildings. The site includes most of the foundations of a large second-century town public bath. There is a major feature of the Jewry Wall which is shared by the basilica.

Littlecote, Wiltshire, England: The bathhouses here are located in Littlecote Park about 3.2 km north-west of Hungerford. The site has three suites of baths and a further part-built bath.

Llandrindod Wells, Powys, Mid Wales: the spa here, with iron, sulphur-rich, and saline waters, claims to have links back to Romano-British times when it is said that the springs were known as Balneae Silures. The best-known Roman settlement in the area was at nearby Castell Collen, which was located just outside Llandrindod Wells. This important archaeological site gives credence to the claims of longevity in the fame of the healing waters here. The local springs were probably known to the Romans but their more recent fame stems from the seventeenth century as the saline springs and other waters became more notable. The major development into the modern spa town was very late, from the mid-1800s onwards.

In fact the popularity of the spas here dropped around the early nineteenth century, in part owing to the reputation of the sumptuous hotel that had been built as a place of anything but healthy relaxation and curative waters. It was the place that the young males of the English aristocracy came in pursuit of what was described as 'debauched dissipation'. As a consequence the hotel was demolished and the town went into a recession for several decades. However, by the end of the 1800s, around 90,000 people *per annum* were visiting and the town boasted two Assembly Rooms, a Pavilion, a Pump Room, and thirty or so mineral wells supplying saline, chalybeate, and sulphur waters.

Lullingstone, Kent, England: The ruins are to be found about 1.6 km west of Eynsford at the end of a side-road from the A225. The centre has a display of archaeological finds and interpretation. The site is of an unusual villa and has late second-century baths which have a long narrow *caldarium* with piers rather than *pilae*. The floors were raised some time during the late fourth century.

Lydney, Gloucestershire, England: The bathhouse here is part of a temple complex and healing sanctuary built towards the end of the fourth century AD.

Matlock, Derbyshire, England: Despite considerable evidence for Matlock being an important Romano-British site on account of its long-established lead smelting, there is nothing to suggest a spa or watering place at that time. There may have been a bathhouse associated with the industries and the settlements in the area, but it is not known today. In the Victorian period, Matlock became a well-known tourism destination with Matlock Bath being closely associated with cold-water hydrotherapy.

Milton Keynes, Buckinghamshire, England: As a 1970s 'new town' it is easy to forget that Milton Keynes includes sites of antiquity. Bancroft Villa is situated in open land just south of Miller's Way and the reconstructed foundations include a bathhouse.

Newport, Isle of Wight, England: The baths are located on Avondale Road and there are displays and a guidebook. The remains include a good suite of baths as part of a second-century winged-corridor villa. There are mosaics *in situ* and well preserved.

North Leigh, Oxfordshire, England: The site is 5 km off the A4095 just north-east of Witney. The remains include a suite of baths associated with a large courtyard villa and earlier baths outlines in gravel.

Orpington, Greater London (Kent), England: The site, situated off Poverest Road, St Mary Cray, Orpington, is the remains of a small Romano-British bathhouse perhaps from the third century AD, and an Anglo-Saxon Cemetery. The bathhouse was excavated between 1971 and 1975 and appears to have been in use from around AD 100. It was extended around AD 270 and became disused about AD 400. The nearby pagan Anglo-Saxon graves are from AD 450 to AD 550.

Portchester, Hampshire, England: Portchester Castle is a stone keep and bailey fortress built in one corner of the Roman fort of Portus Adurni and is located in the town centre off Castle Street, 18 km south-east of Southampton, on the A27. The tall Norman keep stands at the angle of the fort, with a square gatehouse and one square tower flanking the curtain wall. Excavations reveal that despite major defensive structures and especially the massive fortress wall, there was little of significance within the protected area. Most of the barracks buildings were of timber and the only exception was the stone-built bathhouse.

Ravenglass, Cumbria, England: The fort here, called Glanoventa, was built by General Julius Agricola around AD 79. Agricola's progress north was described as being via the 'wooded estuaries', in other words west along the Rivers Lune, Leven, Duddon and Esk, and so up to the Solway Firth. The Ravenglass location for a strategically placed fort was linked to the good harbour and the situation about halfway along the coastline between Morecambe Bay and the Solway. The original structures were timber and turf, replaced about fifty years later by solid buildings of local granite. The bathhouse at Ravenglass is to be found at the end of a long well-wooded drive from the small coastal village nearby. Water was piped to the fort and the bathhouse in lead pipes supplied from a reservoir in woodland higher up the hill that today overlooks the small town of Ravenglass. The remains include well-preserved upstanding walls of the extramural bathhouse for the adjacent Roman fort. Indeed, built around AD 300, the bathhouse is the highest standing Roman ruin in northern Britain. There are internal renderings, a wall niche, and window splays. The fort was used from the first century AD until the fifth century.

Ribchester, Lancashire, England: The village of Ribchester is on the B6245 north of Blackburn. The bathhouse is behind the White Bull public house and the baths are the second-century baths for the associated Roman fort.

Richborough, Kent, England: The baths are associated with a fort on the Kentish 'Saxon Shore' today located on a minor road off the A257 north of Sandwich. The remains lie above the earlier ruins of a *mansio* or posting station.

Rockbourne, Hampshire, England: This site is located 3 km west from Fordingbridge off the A354 and B3078 with a small museum and display boards. Archaeological excavations of the site have been recorded and back-filled for protection, but mosaics and hypocausts are visible. The locations of wall remains are marked by gravel and the post-holes from the buildings are marked. There are two sets of baths with the north-western having *pilae* made from *imbrices* (Roman roof-tiles). The other bathhouses have mosaics and a cold bath.

Segedunum, Wallsend, Northumberland, England: This visitor centre is located on Buddle Street south of the A187 and is a modern full-sized model bathhouse which is an exact replica of the Roman baths at Chesters. The site is designed to give the visitor a real feel for a suite of working baths.

Verulamium, Hertfordshire, England: This was a major Roman town with splendid buildings and structures. The ruins here are the remains of a bath suite from a second-century town house at St Albans. The structures of the *tepidarium* of a bathhouse were discovered by an excavator and are now displayed nearby and include remarkable and intact mosaic floors and a substantial hypocaust system.

Vindolanda, Chesterholme, Northumberland, England: Two military bathhouses are on display about 1 km west of Housteads car park off the B8316. They are a late first-century site to the south outside the stone fort and an early third-century bath to the north-west. Within the site there are also two suites of baths for the commanders of the fort.

Wall, Staffordshire, England: The rather elaborate baths at Wall were part of a *mansio* situated just off what is now the A5 near Brownhills. The hypocaust area has been in-filled and turfed over.

Welwyn, Hertfordshire, England: This site is approached from the Welwyn bypass and is a suite of baths from a third-century villa complex, today protected by a steel vault under the A1(M) embankment. There is a cold room and hot and cold baths.

Witcombe, Gloucestershire, England: The site is approached by a long driveway south of the A417 and east of the A46. There is a well-preserved villa with two suites of baths including a multi-period complex that is now partially covered by modern buildings. The archaeology includes a naïve mosaic of sea animals and a nicely preserved hypocaust now covered by a protective roof.

Wroxeter, Shropshire, England: The remains here include one of the biggest sections of upstanding Roman masonry in the whole of Britain with a huge second-century bathhouse. This wall is called the 'Old Work', bounds the basilica, and is comparable in scale with the Jewry Wall in Leicester.

York, North Yorkshire, England: York's Roman Baths are well worth a visit and are situated in the unusual location of the cellars of a public house, the aptly named Roman Bath Inn. The inn is on Church Street in York and the remains were formerly visible through a glass panel in the saloon bar. Today the baths are open as a small museum to show *caldarium* with *pilae* bases and a section of the tiled *frigidarium* from the fourth-century baths.

This list is by no means complete and certainly omits many sacred springs and wells. However, it does provide a basis for an overview of the main known sites of Roman baths and certainly of those which can be visited by the curious tourist or researcher. Some of these locations are essentially ruins and others are mostly spas and health resorts from a much later period, but with generally tenuous links back to Roman associations. Towns like Buxton are still today famed for their spa waters and certainly had important Roman connections, but these are not visible now. Only Bath, the main site of Romano-British bathing excellence, still maintains its visible links to the Roman baths and the Classical traditions of bathing.

6

DECLINE & FALL

As the Roman Empire fell into ruin, the practice of bathing ended. It is even thought that by bringing malaria from North Africa right into the heart of Rome, the aqueducts, as breeding grounds for mosquitoes, may have hastened the end. By the early fifth century the Roman Empire was beginning to crumble as wave after wave of invaders tried to breach the once impregnable defences. In AD 378, a Germanic people known as the Visigoths defeated the Imperial army at Adrianople, and in AD 408 they marched southwards into Italy itself. Their leader was a noble called Alaric and he had once commanded Gothic troops in the Roman Imperial army. By AD 410, they had entered the City of Rome, becoming the first aggressive force to so do for 800 years. Rome was not sacked since these invaders were Christians and paid great respect to the important churches and similar buildings. However, even when the occupying troops withdrew, the Roman confidence was seriously dented. Within fifty years, a further wave of marauders was on the threshold of Rome as Attila the Hun led his warlike followers through Italy, but he was diverted by a meeting with Pope Leo, and the City was safe. Soon however, the Vandals, another Germanic tribe, arrived via Spain and North Africa, again to pillage and sack the City. Some of the Roman heritage survived but the repeated attacks and the ignominy of such bitter and humiliating defeats sapped the Roman culture and the impacts resonated across all that had formerly been the great empire. Remote yet once-prosperous outposts such as Britain were especially affected and exposed.

Roman bathhouses and bathing cultures were transformed as the ancient Roman Imperial cultures ended and emerged again through Christian and Islamic influences in the Mediterranean and the Middle East. Since

Roman civilisation maintained its political structures and integrity longer and more effectively in the eastern provinces, the culture of baths and bathing continued longer there. Great bathhouses were still being built in Byzantine centres such as Constantinople (modern-day Istanbul) and Antioch. In Italy and Western Europe, the facilities and the practice of bathing went into a rapid decline. In the East, Constantine the Great had inherited the city which straddles Europe and Asia at the Bosphorus and made it his 'New Rome'. Early in the fifth century AD, the city already had eight *thermae* and 153 smaller baths. The Severan Baths of Kaminia were so big that around two thousand people could bathe daily and the bathhouse was noted for its splendid beauty and lighting with abundant naphtha lamps. One of the greatest and oldest baths in the city of Byzas burnt down in AD 432.

Across the former Roman Empire there was a general downturn in the fortunes of baths and bathing from the seventh and eight centuries AD. In the western areas, it was sooner and sharper because of the massive social, political and economic changes that were wrought by the collapse of the Empire. The main difficulty for the bathhouses at this time of invasion and unrest was not that the actual structures of the baths collapsed, but that the aqueduct-borne water supplies did. Very few of the major *thermae* could maintain their water supplies through the period leading up to and through what is often described as the 'Dark Ages', with invasions, political strife, economic downturn and instability. The great baths were technically demanding structures and expensive to maintain. The most troublesome feature however was undoubtedly the complex water supply and water management systems. As Roman cultures were displaced by less sophisticated invaders like the Goths, Vandals, Lombards and others in Europe, and Saxons and then Norse in Britain, the baths were abandoned and the bathhouses fell into dilapidated ruins. In Britain, the tendency was for the incoming Saxons to avoid the larger Roman cities anyway, and to establish new centres. Whilst in the East the bathing cultures survived to an extent, in the Christian-dominated West the broadly based social culture of baths and bathing came to an abrupt end. It was never again to re-emerge in the classical manner and style once the Western Roman Empire had fallen.

Christianity tended to have a negative view of baths, of bathing and especially of bathhouses. Indeed, the early Christian Church discouraged bathing as a pagan pastime and ritual, summed up by the fourth-century ascetic Saint Jerome with 'he who has bathed in Christ has no need of a second bath!' Baths and bathing became caught up in religious rhetoric between Christians and pagans, and between Western and Eastern Christianity. However, despite the disapproval of the great public baths, in centres such as Rome itself, the Western Popes did maintain their own luxurious baths in their palaces and for their own use. Some even built new bathhouses. Furthermore, the Church, never slow to see a business opportunity, realised that bathhouses could make good money. Because of the association of the old bathhouses with pagan rituals, in some cases they had to be exorcised before they could be put to good Christian use. With this in mind, the Diocletian *thermae* in Rome were purified to cleanse their demons before a part of the site was converted into a monastery in the eleventh century.

Early Medieval evidence shows that baths might be incorporated into church buildings or those of monasteries, known as 'charity baths' because they served both the clerics and the needy poor. Overindulgence, especially hot baths, could bring criticism and censure, but behind closed doors, those in high office still enjoyed these luxuries. The problem with bathing for devout Christians was not so much the bath itself but the clash with the idea of achieving spirituality by enduring physical and bodily deprivation. Because bathing was pleasurable as well as functional, this troubled the devout adherent. So it was acceptable for the masses to bathe, as long as they didn't enjoy it.

This attitude was summed up succinctly by Barsanuphius, a hermit from Palestine: 'Bathing is not absolutely forbidden to one who needs it. If you are ill you need it; so it is not a sin. If a man is healthy, it cossets and relaxes the body and conduces to lust.' Similarly, Pope Gregory the Great (AD 540–604) stated that baths are 'for the needs of the body … not for the titillation of the mind and sensuous pleasure'.

In this vein many thermal baths and healing spas continued to function throughout the period. The famous and sometimes infamous spa city of Baiae, as noted earlier, continued in use until the seventeenth century. Whilst its use through this time was as a healing and medicinal centre, the sensuality of its earlier times and Seneca's assessment of the city as a 'resort of vice' were never quite erased. The Christian Church could tolerate medicinal bathing but not the pleasurable hot springs of a recreational resort which might titillate the body and lead to lust. Indeed some Christian writers considered that thermal spas were the places 'where the devil himself sets his snares because men and women bathe together.' Specifically, the old-fashioned gymnasia and indeed gymnastics were strongly disapproved of. The latter harked back to the Greek imagery of naked gymnasts and was too much for emerging Christianity to cope with.

As cults such as *alousa* developed, named in this case after the ascetic ideal of being unwashed, the idea of being dirty emerged as a spiritually good thing; it emphasised the spiritual triumph over the body. Furthermore, it stressed the singular importance of baptism as the only true and valid form of bathing 'in Christ'. The followers were mainly monks, priests and hermits, and they sought spiritual godliness by avoiding personal hygiene. This is some way from the more modern concept that 'cleanliness is next to godliness'! Perhaps they smelled to high heaven.

So whilst some baths and cultures of bathing remained in the East, public bathing by the masses fell dramatically after the collapse of the Roman Empire in the West in AD 476. Three or four centuries followed that we often describe as the Dark Ages. Some bathhouses remained and the practice of bathing continued for some, but these were mainly the privileged few. In the northern countries such as Britain, it is likely that bathing was reduced to a very few exceptional situations such as specific healing spas and springs. However, a remarkable re-emergence was about to happen and perhaps this fulfilled all the worst expectations of the Christian ascetics.

There are richly decorated illustrations from medieval manuscripts showing pairs of wooden bath-tubs with couples, men and women, feasting, drinking and carousing. The couples face each other over wooden boards on which a white linen runner is placed and food is laid out. The couples are naked apart from headwear and jewellery and attendants offer food, drink, music and more. A room to one side shows a separate room where a couple, again naked, are going to bed. The bedchamber appears to be a part of the offering of the facility and the whole image, whilst not openly lewd, is very suggestive. The presence in the image of a senior figure with a crown and sceptre suggests royalty, and the interpretation is that this bathhouse offers far more then cleanliness. This is a far cry from the post-Roman ascetics, the facility luxurious but sleazy. There are many illustrations and descriptions of mixed communal bathing in medieval times and most have a sensual element to them. The suggestion is that the baths were a centre for illicit liaisons and even for prostitution. These depictions perhaps exaggerate the licentiousness and it is likely that other bathhouses had opened to offer basic pleasant bathing in hot water and pleasant surroundings. The facilities also offered barbers, doctors, depilators and masseurs to service a broad base of often working clientèle.

Bathing was quick to become popular in the German regions north of the Alps, and it was maintained there for longer as the bathhouses closed and plague swept across Europe. The Germanic bathers were also more casual about nudity than their equivalents in southern Europe. An Italian doctor living in Germany during the 1400s described how this began even with the walk from home to the bathhouse, when entire families including adolescent children would walk naked or near-naked through the town on their way to bathe. As a result of complaints to the authorities, laws were enacted to bring more decorum to the streets, but the extent to which they had an effect is not clear.

It is likely that such bathhouses were more common in southern continental Europe, particularly Italy and France, and in parts of Germany, than they were in Britain. Paris by 1292 had a population of around 70,000 people served by twenty-six public baths. These included 'steam baths' which had been a speciality in the *laconicum* of Roman baths though its origins were most likely amongst the semi-nomadic peoples of the great European steppes of Russia. The heating performed by the hypocaust in Roman baths was mostly replaced by the simple heating of a cauldron of water over furnaces located in a basement. Some more sophisticated systems were used including quite extravagant structures resembling large distillation vessels, but these were not common. Occasionally in the most grand of mansions or palaces, such as the residence of the Pope at Avignon, or the Dukes of Brittany at Suscinio, there might be a two-room bathing suite with under-floor hypocaust heating, but this was very rare. Generally, one room would have tubs for bathing and the other would be a steam room. Water was occasionally piped in from a distant source, but mostly it relied on servants and buckets rushing to and fro from a nearby well or river.

It may be that the resurgence of interest and enjoyment in Britain and Western Europe was in part due to the returning Crusaders. Having experienced the luxuries of Eastern living, they wanted to bring this habit of bathing back home. To a more significant degree than in the West, as described earlier, the Roman bathing traditions had persisted longer in the Eastern Mediterranean. This renewal of interest and acceptance in the West seems to have coincided with an upsurge in public enjoyment of personal hygiene and also in the sensuous delights of the bathhouse. However, by the fifteenth century the bathhouses, at least in cities such as London, had become synonymous with brothels, many run for the economy and benefit of the Church. Lordly private baths were already known as places of assignation but the growing public bathhouses soon established a dual function. These were facilities where ordinary citizens, respectable people with their children, would go to bathe, but where prostitutes would also operate. Patrons would go to bathe in steam and hot water but also would order food, wine, and if necessary, compliant serving girls. The 'stews' or 'stewhouses' grew from being places of public bathing to being synonymous with houses of prostitution. It seems that so long as this did not inconvenience or threaten the regular customers, then it was considered a legitimate side-line of the business. Indeed, in fifteenth-century France for example, there was little or no shame attached to visiting prostitutes and the bathhouse became what was later called a 'bawdy house' or *maison de tolérance*, and of a somewhat higher class than the basic brothels. In England, by the twelfth century, Henry II recognised the Southwark area of London, with its stews, as a formal red-light district. However, as the risk of public disorder and the spread of diseases such as syphilis began to cause concerns, the authorities started to take actions to control the stews. London Council attempted to ban all stews except those owned privately for the purposes of cleanliness. This had little effect until the sixteenth century as diseases including plague spread and the stews were deemed responsible.

Despite this burgeoning interest and the great profitability of the public baths, things were about to change as a new moral code swept through Europe. The increased sexual freedom and the liberating atmosphere of the bathhouse were gradually associated with the insidious spread of sexually transmitted diseases. Whilst the precise history of rise of syphilis is still debated, there is no doubt that in the 1500s it swept through Europe to devastating effect. For a variety of reasons an especially virulent form of the disease spread from Italy to France, then Germany and England. The effects were debilitating, grotesquely unpleasant, and often deadly. This dramatic turn of events gave the conservative and Reformist lobbies a tangible reason to close down the public baths. In France, Germany, and England, orders were given for the prohibition of public bathhouses and brothels; the only exceptions were a few of the better-known thermal healing spas. In England Henry VIII famously closed the London stews, but probably not before he himself had been infected with syphilis. The precise mode of spread was unknown because there was only very limited knowledge of the mechanisms of disease. Hot on the heels of the syphilitic outbreak there followed bubonic plague, which also devastated urban populations across Western Europe and Britain. Medical opinion of the time believed that plague was associated with close social contact and therefore the bathhouses were once again suspect. A statement which summed up the general belief was 'bathhouses and steam-baths, I beg you, flee from them or you shall die!'

This fear played up to a deep-seated misunderstanding of how the human body functioned. Health was related to the balance of the so-called 'humours' and illness was the manifestation of an imbalance. Furthermore, physicians believed that the human skin functioned as a permeable membrane and that its pores, if not protected by dirt, were open to the influx of disease and infection. With this view in mind, the idea of bathing in a hot steamy atmosphere could be tantamount to suicide. The soapy water, the steam and the relaxation would allow the body to be penetrated by deadly infection and so any such bathing activity was to be rigorously avoided. Indeed, if bathing was recommended for other health reasons, it was only to be undertaken with strict medical supervision. 'Bath-houses and steam-baths will from now on be deserted, because the pores and the little air holes in the skin, being as a result of the heat, more easily opened, foul air gets in' (Hovel, 1573 in Yegül, 2010). In many ways, these beliefs echoed the fears from classical times about hot baths weakening and softening the constitution. In some situations however, cold-water bathing could be used, and according to certain medical opinions, to good effect.

The attitudes to bathing affected the perceptions and fears of water more generally. The latter became regarded as something inherently dangerous and bad for both the body and for good health. It was acceptable and safe to 'view' water in fountains, pools, and cascades in grand and beautiful estates, but it was only to be enjoyed at a distance. The idea of water as a cleansing and purifying agent good for health was banished across Western Europe. Even bathing in private was reduced to a simple wiping of the face with a damp cloth. Occasionally for personal hygiene reasons the body might be wiped as well, but this would not be a common occurrence. More likely a scented linen cloth, the so-called 'dry wash', would be used in preference to water. Cleanliness was regarded as a matter of fresh clean linen and this itself became a cleansing act. Fashion and cleanliness became closely aligned; but it was cleanliness in the absence of close contact with water. You could be 'clean' without washing but with fresh linen and perfume.

This new emergence of an antipathy for water was in many ways similar to that of the early Christian ascetics and the Christian ideal of being 'unwashed'. By the seventeenth and eighteenth centuries, private houses, including the most luxurious premises, would have virtually no faculties for washing beyond a silver bowl and pitcher in which to wash one's hands. Furthermore, there may well have been a distaste for bathing and baths as they were now associated strongly with Eastern and Islamic living and influences. Long-standing links to the Roman classical ideas of bathhouses and bathing were now effectively severed. Certainly in cold northern climes such as Britain, and during the several centuries of what is known as the 'Little Ice Age', bathing, publicly or privately, was banished. Baths were strongly associated in the public mind with serious threats to health, and to moral and sexual degradation allied to pagan and Islamic rituals. The only exceptions would be a few healing spas and perhaps religiously significant springs. By the end of the sixteenth century, bathing was considered to be a thoroughly dead practice. King James I of England supposedly only ever washed his fingers, and Henri IV of France was notoriously smelly, his son, Louis XIII, stating how 'I take after my father, I smell of armpits'.

Personal hygiene and cleanliness were really at a long-term low with most people avoiding exposure to, or contact with, water. This was then reflected in all sorts of manifestations from body odour to halitosis. Even the rich and famous were not immune to such things. King Louis XIV of France for example, the great 'Sun King', was also notable for his bad breath and his mistress Madame de Montespan complained bitterly and swathed herself under clouds of strong perfumes. Writers of the time were also bemused by Turkish cultures where people bathed several times a week and even washed their genitals. This was considered exotic and bizarre. Even Madame de Montespan, who was so offended by the King's bad breath, was herself described by her attendants as being visibly dirty when viewed naked.

The poor people of the time, lacking public baths of any description, would also be dirty and smelly. A combination of lack of resources and medical opinions would deny access to water or cleansing to most people. The whole problem of hygiene was endemic and the presence of fleas and lice in hair and wigs of all from the highest to the lowest in society is well-known. In eighteenth-century Baden in Switzerland, the ladies were noted for carrying great numbers of fleas in the ringlets of their hair or of their wigs. Their escorts or partners would have the apparently delightful task of picking the fleas off their pale white skin. An anonymous text, the 'Book of Amusements', described how 'in young women, dancing produces a surprising effect. As soon as they begin to perspire freely, fleas emerge from their ringlets, causing a certain amount of distress. As these women have such beautiful skins, it is a pleasurable duty to pick off the vermin as soon as they appear.'

7

RUINS & ROMANTICS

However, by the 1600s and 1700s, attitudes to water, to health and to personal hygiene were beginning to change. This was to be reflected in personal behaviour and also in what were adopted as social norms. The fear of water and the disapproval of baths and bathing were to be put to one side and new fashions of spa visiting and of hygiene and water therapy would emerge.

As the medieval period ended, the Roman ruins began to acquire a 'Romantic' appeal to poets and writers keen to touch a past link to philosophers and writers from classical times. As Europe and Britain emerged from the Renaissance and into the modern era, there was a tendency to look back to the classics, to Rome and to Greece. Long-abandoned Romano-British ruins began to acquire a new significance and interest. Throughout the period when baths and bathing were both essentially outlawed, curative baths for the sick and thermal bathing and spas were still allowed. Taking a bath would however be under strict medical and religious supervision. This was a dangerous process not to be undertaken lightly. The famous thermal spas and baths were at Aquae Sulis (in Bath), England, at Vichy in France, at Baden-Baden and Wiesbaden, in Germany, and Baiae in Italy. Here, the sick would visit to take the waters and to seek relief or even cures for their maladies. Instruction and association harked back to the writings of Roman doctors, and the wealthy arrived with their private physicians whilst the middle classes used the advisers on hand at the spa itself. In times of limited medical understanding or treatment for the sick, these few centres not only kept their doors open, but they thrived.

Interestingly, the poorer classes throughout this period, whilst often dressed in rags, probably made more use of bathing in rivers, lakes and even the sea, than did their affluent social superiors. They would be more concerned with the practicalities of mundane day-to-day living and working than the adherence to the pronouncements of physicians and philosophers. Mud and grime from daily working would be washed off under the village pump or in the local stream.

Then, in Europe in particular, there was a great change following the death in France of the Sun King, Louis XIV in 1715. With a move in high society back to the cities, there began a reawakening of interest in the pleasures and benefits of bathing and the public bathhouse. What had recently been a fearful and dangerous practice quickly grew to be a mark of good taste and sophistication. From the late seventeenth century and into the eighteenth century, the fashion of real 'cleanliness' and the urbanite delights of the sensual and sexual pleasures of the bathhouse grew to become a public craze. Baths were established along rivers such as the Seine in France and catered for everything from the urban poor to the pampered aristocracy. There was also a resurgence in the idea of swimming too. Riverside bathhouses offered cleansing facilities but also showers, massage, hair removal and more. Wealthy patrons could eat and drink, with feasts including truffles in champagne, lamb seared and cooked in tomatoes, and more. The Bains Tivoli offered a prenuptial bath experience during which the bridegroom could be massaged with Peruvian clove balm, vanilla, and cinnamon together with a special crushed insect reputed to be an aphrodisiac. Bathing facilities were offered for men and women, and increasingly there was a mock-Oriental style to the décor and there would be musical entertainment too. The whole experience seemed to hark back to the grandeur of the greatest Roman *thermae* of classical times.

In the wider realms of society there was renewed interest in Classical influences and styles. This was a period of great landscaped parks and gardens, and sumptuous halls, houses and palaces located within them. Ancient ruins gave a patina of antiquity and elegance to newly built houses, and links to Roman times were particularly prized. If the estate did not include a Roman ruin, then of course one could be built as a folly. With the emergence of the Romantic Movement in Europe, and especially in Britain, the fashionable elegance of buildings, landscapes, historic sites, and Classical romantic ruins became of paramount importance. Some wealthy landowners even built mock Roman baths as a part of their elegant romantic estate. Again, with the increasing trend of spending a part of the year on your estate and a part in London or some other fashionable resort, the romantic associations of the newly rediscovered Roman baths in Bath acquired a new magnetism.

Across Europe too, the wealthy and fashionable British would go on their Grand Tours to absorb culture. Across continental Europe and into the Mediterranean, these bright young things of British society would see and acquire a taste for all things Classical, Romantic, and even Oriental. The ideas and aspirations were then transported back to the British Isles to impact on a new fashion and taste for baths, bathing and Classical culture. A new significance was attached to ancient cultures and Roman ruins, and to the ideals and images of Italian sophistication, architecture and art.

Sacred healing wells, springs and spas which had survived the downturn in attitudes to water, would quickly re-acquire a new significance. Healing waters and curative powers would gain a new importance as urban populations still struggled with endemic diseases and the possibility, just as in Roman times, of sudden and inexplicable death. Sacred waters linked to miracles and increasingly, spas and therapies based on a mix of science and pseudo-science, would draw and attract desperate and gullible sufferers from illness. Furthermore, there was a rapidly increasing market for the sensual and other delights of the baths and the bathhouses. If it was possible to mix all these elements together at a particular location, then this was a recipe for future success and prosperity.

However, a transformation in facilities, services and environments would be required. When Nash (see Chapter 8) arrived at Bath for example, he discovered it to be 'one of the poorest cities in England' and as a nameless magazine writer stated, it was 'a scruffy minor spa of squalid lodgings, roving ruffians and pick-pockets, quack doctors and nude bathing in unhygienic public baths by visitors whose principle employments were yawning and drinking those waters which nothing but the most extraordinary fear of death … could ever have reconciled any human being to touching after the first drop' (in Searle, 1977). The influence of Nash in particular was to transform Bath into the most beautiful, formalised, and meticulously managed spa anywhere in the world.

By 1790, Horace Walpole was able to observe that 'one would think the English were ducks; they are for ever waddling to the waters'.

8

THE RE-EMERGENCE OF BATHS & SPAS

Alongside a new romantic awareness was a re-emergence of the idea of bathing and health. Bearing in mind that many medical practitioners believed that contact with water was damaging, and immersion in water could be life-threatening and was to be undertaken only with medical supervision, this was revolutionary stuff. However, in a society struck down by many diseases associated with increased urban living, people were desperate for something to ease their suffering. Attending a spa, and at least being clean, obviously helped. Across Europe, especially in Germany and associated countries there was a boom in health spas and health spa visiting. This new fashion spilled over into Britain and was to last up until the 1930s, after which the bathing and spa culture declined once more, only to pick up again in the late twentieth century.

Of the four main spa centres in post-Reformation seventeenth-century England, only one, Bath, owed its presence to earlier healing waters. The others were based on waters more recently discovered: Harrogate in Yorkshire (1571), Epsom in Surrey (1618), and Tunbridge in Kent (1606). There were of course others, but these four make up the core of the early spas which left a significant legacy to modern times. Sites such as Astrop in Oxfordshire (patronised by Celia Fiennes) and the Clifton Hot Wells in the Severn Gorge near Bristol, also enjoyed short-lived fame and fortune. Barnet near London for a while became a spa town and was frequented by clients such as Samuel Pepys. In London itself there were of course centres whose names live on today, such as Sadler's Wells, and spas at Islington, Clerkenwell, and Sydenham. Some of these died out as spas but grew as entertainment and leisure centres.

A key to the development of these seventeenth-century spa centres was the discovery of their remarkable healing waters. Early in the seventeenth century, so-called chalybeate water was said to have health-giving and curative medicinal properties; many authorities of the time promoting its special qualities. Spas and wells associated with such waters began to spring up across England. In 1606, Dudley North, Third Baron North, discovered a chalybeate spring at Tunbridge Wells and his physician claimed that the waters containing 'vitriol' would cure: 'the colic, the melancholy, and the vapours; it made the lean fat, the fat lean; it killed flat worms in the belly, loosened the clammy humours of the body, and dried the over-moist brain.' The well-known English physician Thomas Sydenham prescribed chalybeate waters for problems such as 'hysteria': 'These waters youth in age renew Strength to the weak and sickly and Give the pale cheek a rosy hue And cheerful spirits to the sad.'

The origins of the word 'chalybeate' are from the Latin word for steel: *chalybs*. This derives from the Greek word *khalups*, the singular form of the *Khalubes* or *Chalybes*, the name of a mythical people living on Mount Ida in northern Asia Minor and who supposedly invented iron working. 'Ferruginous' is from the Latin word *ferreus* which means 'made of iron' and comes from the Latin word *ferrum*, literally 'iron'.

The chalybeate waters from Tunbridge Wells were analysed in 1967 and shown to contain (parts per million):

Iron (II) carbonate: $FeCO_3$	25.3 ppm
Manganese (II) carbonate: $MnCO_3$	4.6 ppm
Calcium sulphate: $CaSO_4$	60.9 ppm
Magnesium sulphate: $MgSO_4$	13.4 ppm
Magnesium chloride: $MgCl_2$	7.8 ppm
Sodium chloride: NaCl	57.2 ppm
Potassium chloride: KCl	7.3 ppm

Once the fashion for these curative waters was established, physicians and entrepreneurs scoured the countryside, anxious to find healing waters and tourism honey-pots. A somewhat ornate spring well is to be found in the village of Quarndon in Derbyshire with a plaque inside the well bearing the following description '17th century chalybeate spring well. Once famous spa noted for medicinal waters containing iron. Visited by Daniel Defoe in 1727'. The well is on the roadside just down from the Joiners' Arms public house. The iron-rich waters made this a popular watering place long before the growth of Harrogate or Matlock Bath, but its waters stopped following an earth tremor in 1817, and the well was last decorated in the year 2000. The waters were said to be 'specific in Coughs, Asthma, Consumption,

Spittin of blood, Hyppa and Cachexy'; they also warded off plague. This was typical of the sorts of discoveries and claims for healing made to a desperate and gullible population. Another spring was at Bermondsey, south-east of the Tower of London, where, around 1770, Thomas Keyse opened tea gardens and following the discovery of a chalybeate spring, the gardens became known as Bermondsey Spa. In 1784, Keyse got a licence to 'provide in his garden musical entertainments' like those in the Vauxhall Pleasure Gardens, plus occasional exhibitions of fireworks. The admission price was one shilling.

Some of the better-known English chalybeate springs included the following: Alexandra Park in Hastings, East Sussex; Bermondsey Spa, London; Chalice Well, Glastonbury; Cheltenham, Gloucestershire; Chalybeate Kennels near Ingleborough, North Yorkshire; Dorton Spa, Dorton, Buckinghamshire; The Gloucester Spa, Gloucester; Griffydam, Leicestershire; Hampstead, North London; Harrogate, North Yorkshire; Kedleston Hall, Quarndon, Derbyshire; Kilburn, North London; Lees, Greater Manchester; Nill Well, between Yelling and Papworth Everard, Cambridgeshire; St Ann's Well Gardens, Hove, East Sussex; St Blaise's Well, Bromley, Kent; Seend, Wiltshire; Somersham, Cambridgeshire; Sandrock Spring, Isle of Wight; Southwick, Northamptonshire; Tunbridge Wells, Kent; and Winteringham, North Lincolnshire.

Other spas, including Harrogate, also boasted strongly sulphurous waters with additional impacts on health, and especially on taste. Some locations had saline waters alongside the iron-rich chalybeate, the sulphur springs and the peat or mud baths.

Harrogate was one of the most remarkable stories of the growth of a major and still today thriving centre, from absolutely nothing. Within a couple of centuries the town was the 'first English Spaw' and also known as the 'spa on the desolate moors'. The waters were found in the sixteenth century by William Slingsby, and it was he who realised the close resemblance of the waters to those of Spa in Germany. He had been there as a soldier during the Continental Wars, and was quick to spot the potential of his discovery. Then, in 1596, Timothy Bright, a local physician, published a tract in praise of the curative waters of Harrogate. At first, the main beneficiary of the attraction of the waters was in fact the much older and wealthier town of Knaresborough, and Harrogate remained just a huddle of poor cottages on a bleak, windswept moor. Gradually however, the facilities around Harrogate itself grew and improved, and visitors spent 'the season' there. Outside the season, they still stayed in Knaresborough.

Many genuine and sometimes quack physicians published books, pamphlets and guides to the waters and the places. A physician, Doctor Anthony Relhan (*c.* 1715–76), for example, promoted the drinking of mineral waters. He was especially impressed by the healing waters from the chalybeate spring in St Anne's Well Gardens in Hove, and published 'A Short History of Brighthelmstone; with Remarks on its Air, an Analysis of its Waters, Particularly of an uncommon Mineral one, long discovered, though but lately used in 1761'. Many such books were produced and became overnight best-sellers. The books led to a significant upsurge in popular interest in both bathing in and drinking mineral waters. Following the publicity a grateful public might heap praise and reward on the discoverer. In this case, the American town of Enfield in New Hampshire changed its name, albeit temporarily, to Relhan in honour of the great man and his Sussex therapy.

At nearby Tunbridge Wells in 1834, Princess Victoria, soon to be Queen Victoria, drank the waters every day during her stay in the town. Victoria, with mother, the Duchess of Kent, would visit the spring and then enjoy a stroll along the Pantiles, the pretty, colonnaded walkway which is the most well-known aspect of what is now Royal Tunbridge Wells. The area was formerly the playground of gentry and royalty, associated with the discovery of the Chalybeate Spring in the early seventeenth century. The subsequent popularity of the spa water amongst fashionable Georgian gentry and the royalty triggered the growth of Tunbridge Wells as a spa resort. In the eighteenth century, the area surrounding the famous spring was developed as a colonnaded walkway, later known as 'The Pantiles'. The 'Walks' became the place for visitors to see and be seen. With a strict protocol, gentry paraded on the colonnaded 'Upper Walks' and the lesser visitors enjoyed the 'Lower Walks'. During 'the season' the self-appointed Master of Ceremonies, Richard Beau Nash, a fashion icon and noted dandy, ensured that this protocol was respectfully adhered to. The water at the heart of this tourism and health boom contains significant levels of dissolved mineral salts and the high concentrations of iron and manganese give it a characteristic flavour.

The waters here were reputed to be good for a whole range of disorders including somewhat undefinable sufferings such as 'melancholia' which seemed to afflict the younger gentry of the time. They also had curative powers for infertility and related problems. In 1630, for example they were visited by Queen Henrietta Maria, consort of King Charles I, and there followed the birth of the later Prince James. The town barely existed and the Queen, with her entourage, were accommodated in tents and temporary wooden buildings. Of the place it was said that 'the Horizon is fill'd with an inexhaustible series of Odoriferous and Fragrant Effluviums', which the royal party seemed to enjoy. King Charles II was another visitor to Tunbridge for its healing waters and to escape the claustrophobic and disease-ridden environs of plague-filled London. Royal patronage of Tunbridge had already given it a reputation for easy living and licentious behaviour such that the Puritans had described the healing wells as 'the waters of scandal'.

Epsom was the most successful of the spas located close to London, but in fact its proximity and ease of access would actually prove its undoing. In 1618, Henry Wicker, a local farmer, was enlarging a watering-hole for his cattle when he found that they would not drink the water that the spring produced. Perplexed, he himself tasted the water and realised that though it might not appeal to bovines, it was certainly good for people. Soon it was claimed that the Epsom waters cured gout, liver complaints and more. With Epsom being so close to London, the small town was soon overwhelmed by visitors desperately seeking cures for their illnesses. In the period after the Restoration, Epsom was patronised by King Charles II and his various mistresses, particularly Nell Gwyn, who would be accommodated at a nearby inn. The diarist Samuel Pepys also stayed at Epsom and he recorded that the waters gave him 'many good stools'. Epsom was so busy that he had to stay at nearby Ashtead. Amusements and activities included gaming, dancing, bowls, wrestling, cudgel-playing and hawking. Horse-racing, which began on the nearby Downs, led to the modern-day 'Derby Week'.

However, Epsom's strength was also its weakness. It was too close to London to be sufficiently exclusive for the more discerning patrons. Overrun by tradesmen and lesser people, the nobility and the royals left, and their places were taken by wealthy middle classes. In the early eighteenth century, the town still received 2,000 visitors a day to take the waters and business was good, though the spa had gone down-market and was no longer a fashionable place to be seen. But worse was to come, as under the unremitting pressure of the masses, the unique healing well ran dry. With a hint of subterfuge, local businessmen, not wishing to risk their livelihoods, began to top the well up from other nearby sites under cover of darkness. These other sources lacked the essential mineral content of the Epsom waters, and the old well was eventually bought and closed down by a Dr John Livingstone. He decided to protect the reputation of the well by preventing further contamination, but then remarkably soon, discovered a new source of the healing waters. His business intervention relaunched the spa town with new assembly rooms and gaming facilities. Indeed, for a short while the new project attracted the patronage of the Prince Regent, George Augustus and of his mistress Mrs Fitzherbert. However, George soon bored of the Oriental bazaar at Epsom and was lured to Brighton by its new Oriental Palace, thus marking the terminal downturn in the fortunes of Epsom. The fashionable visitors flocked to Brighton to follow the Prince Regent, and Epsom lives on in its liver salts, packed and sold to other spa towns and to chemists across the country.

Of the main spa towns of the seventeenth and eighteenth centuries, it was Bath which had genuine roots back to earlier and even to Classical times. Royal patronage was again central to the success of the re-emergence of Bath as a fashionable centre. Anne of Modena, the Queen of James I, King of England, was somewhat slow in producing the heir that was so important in terms of political stability. The advice from the Royal Physician, Sir Theodore Mayerne, was to send her off on a series of visits to the healing waters of Bath. When Anne indeed produced the required heir, then Bath's reputation for solving fertility problems was widely touted by the burgesses of the town. The result seems to have been that the place was inundated with infertile noble-women eagerly seeking the cure.

In many ways, as the thermal waters of Bath began to become popular during the fifteenth century, there was little to suggest that they would reach the dizzy heights of sophistication which they achieved during the seventeenth and eighteenth centuries. In the time of Elizabeth I they became famed for the healing of leprosy and other skins diseases. 'Custom' of the time meant that all bathers took the waters naked and this led to crowds of eager onlookers. If anyone had the nerve to enter the waters semi-clothed then the crowd were not above forcibly stripping them. If a visitor did manage to evade the crowds and their insistence on nude bathing, then they could actually be fined, once more, 'according to custom'. In 1449, in order to address concerns over the rowdy behaviour, the Bishop of Bath and Wells, Thomas Beckington, instructed that all bathers and particularly adolescent girls and boys, were to be 'decorously clad'; the exceptions were children below the age of puberty. However, reports indicate that the Bishop's pronouncements had little effect, and the reputation of Bath as a centre for bawdy riotous behaviour continued. At this early time, the warm waters of Bath were yet to grow into the luxurious attraction for the rich and sickly nobility. However, things would change and develop over the following couple of centuries. The sanitation at Bath, or rather its absence, was also criticised: Elizabeth I was unimpressed when visiting her godson Sir John Harrington who observed that 'their common sewer, which before stood in an ill place, stands now in no place, for they have not any at all; which for a towne so plentifully served of water, in a country so well provided of stone, in a place resorted to so greatly, seemeth an unworthy and dishonourable thing.'

The town boasted five baths of which the most exclusive and private was the King's Bath, which was surrounded by a series of stone arches giving a degree of seclusion from prying eyes. Only the Hot Bath was in part covered from the elements, the others being totally open. Weather and local viewers could make a visit to the baths quite an ordeal, with the local populace not above tricks like throwing a dog over and into the waters, just to liven things up. As in the earlier Roman times, concerns were expressed about whether indeed such bathing of so many people in such close proximity could indeed be hygienic or health-giving. Samuel Pepys in particular expressed concerns over the unhygienic conditions. However, after the Reformation, and with the patronage of King Charles II and his mistresses, the Duchesses of Portland and of Cleveland, the place thrived despite the often squalid conditions. In this rather run-down medieval town, the walls of lodging houses were given a wash of beer and soot to try and disguise the accumulated grime. Out of season the place was deserted and desolate.

Yet by the eighteenth century this would all change and Bath would witness a quite remarkable transformation into a vision created by Palladian architects. The man who is largely credited with bringing about this change was one Richard 'Beau' Nash, mentioned earlier in connection with Tunbridge Wells. He came to Bath as deputy to the man in charge of the town's gaming tables, a man called Captain Webster. Following Webster's demise in a duel following a dispute at the tables, Nash assumed full control; one of his first acts was to banish swords from the gambling rooms. The township over which he assumed a degree of influence and control was a rather mixed bag. There were local gentry and country squires from the neighbourhood, the indigenous poor of the town, the affluent businessmen and well-to-do traders, and then the fashionable visitors. In the socially stratified society of the time, many of these people would normally have little contact with each other. Here in Bath, in the season the low and the high would, however reluctantly, be rubbing shoulders with each other. This was a social melting pot in the same mould as the great Roman *thermae*. The visitors would include the nobility and royalty normally associated with London, rather than with a provincial town. Following these wealthy and influential patrons were huge numbers of gamblers, sportsmen, fortune-hunters and hangers-on, rakes, courtesans and prostitutes, profiteers, speculators, criminals, villains and petty crooks, and the fashion-seeking social butterflies of the age.

Into this cauldron of social melee there was the influence of two very different men. First was Richard Nash, the self-declared arbiter of taste and fashion in Bath as the Master of Ceremonies; secondly there was Ralph Allen, who set about making Bath beautiful. Allen was a Cornishman who had made a fortune from his radical reorganisation of the Royal Mail service. He acquired the land and resources to build the new town, and in Yorkshireman John Wood the Elder, an architect capable of setting out a city in the classical style to be comparable with any in Europe. John Wood died before his vision could be implemented, but the work was carried on and completed by his son, John Wood the Younger.

Ralph Allen provided much of the capital resources to build the great crescents and squares of Bath. Richard Nash however, was the one who directed the leisurely occupations of the people who occupied the properties during the season. He worked tirelessly to organise subscriptions to fund musical entertainments and a playhouse, and to provide public access to parks and walks from which they were previously excluded. He even applied his influence to the town's burgesses in order to get them to pave the major roads into Bath and to organise for their cleaning. This all helped to create the unique atmosphere and pleasurable experience of the season at Bath.

Nash even managed to inject a degree of social politeness and decorum into the society whirlpool which Bath had become. He insisted that troublesome local squires and others were discouraged from loutish behaviour, especially when this was directed at visiting nobility or others of high station. However, he also took to task the higher echelons of society if they were too snobbish towards those of lower social status. For the time, this was a remarkably egalitarian step.

> That gentlemen of fashion never appearing in a morning before ladies in caps or gowns show breeding and respect.
> That no gentleman give his tickets for balls to nay but gentlewomen NB unless he has none of his acquaintance.
> That no gentleman or Lady takes it ill that another dances before them – except such as have no pretence to dance at all.
> That the older ladies and children be content with a second bench at the ball, as being past or not yet come to perfection.
> That a ceremony at coming to Bath, and another at going away, is all that is expected of Ladies of quality and fashion; except impertinents.

> That no person take it ill that anyone goes to another's play, or breakfast, and not theirs – except captious by nature.
> That all whisperers of scandal and lies be taken for their authors.

Above are Beau Nash's 'Rules of Conduct' for visitors to Bath in the early eighteenth century. These were not really rules as such, but more guidance on social etiquette.

THE CURATIVE AND HEALTH-GIVING WATERS

For many centuries, a part of the healing process involved actually visiting the spa and taking the waters there *in situ*. Indeed, to remove the water from its source was somehow to diminish its efficacy. Some of the waters or their salts were certainly taken to centres such as London, but for many people the water separated from its 'life-giving fount' was worthless. By the end of the Victorian age the situation had changed and whilst visiting to take the local waters was good, many facilities boasted a plethora of exotic treatments to suit all tastes. These novel treatments included exotic ideas such as electrotherapy, mud and peat baths, compressed air baths, galvanisation, and a whole range of treatments under the broad term of hydropathy. The spas which remained by the late 1800s and early 1900s offered almost all these treatments under one roof. Whereas the early seeker after healing waters might go from place to place for different ailments and different cures, now you could get them altogether. To some degree this had already happened, with the great spa towns of Harrogate, Cheltenham and Bath offering many different cures and various wells or springs in close proximity.

Hygiene and the mixed (or at least sequential) bathing of the ill and the healthy seem to still have caused concerns in the nineteenth century. A. B. Granville, the author of a major account of English spas published in 1841, described the scene at Buxton:

> When I beheld the class of persons ... who kept coming in (for the access is free and the bath always open) and their dress and appearance – when I saw the pot-bellied farmer of sixty half palsied, and the lame artisan with his black and calloused hands, and the many who suffered from cutaneous disorders – all plunging together, or one after the other, in quick succession – some of whom would set about scrubbing from their hardened cuticles the congregated perspiration of ages ... when I beheld all these things, I confess my courage failed me.

Yet despite this, sufferers from problems such as arthritis flocked to the Buxton thermal baths for a chance of a cure or at least temporary relief.

BATHING IN MUD AND PEAT

One of the therapeutic treatments, which goes back to Roman times and before, was to bathe in hot mud at a thermal spring site. This practice occurs around the world wherever the geological conditions facilitate it. In other locations organic mud from lakes or peat from bogs was used with or instead of the mineral mud. There are numerous mud and peat spas across Eastern Europe and in the United States of America. In Britain, famous peat spas were to be found at Strathpether in Scotland, Harrogate and Buxton in England, and Llandrindod Wells, in mid-Wales. The mud and peat traditions are truly global in extent, and an American example illustrates a process that has occurred in many places all around the world. A famous American spa developed at Waukesha in Wisconsin with the Grand View Resort. John Weber, a Milwaukee real estate agent, had bought an 87-acre plot on the northern side of Waukesha, Wisconsin when he discovered 'black moor mud'. He soon realised that this had similar medicinal properties to deposits in European mud baths and especially the 'black moor mud' of certain German spas. Following a visit to research the German spas and their treatments, he decided to go ahead and build the 'Moor Down Mud Baths' and an associated health resort. This was the Grand View Health Resort, built and opened in 1911, and now part of the Waukesha County Office Buildings. It has also seen time as a Catholic seminary. The original hotel and resort comprised thirty-two rooms with an extension to add a further thirty. In 1919, another local entrepreneur added a golf course surrounding the complex and this is still in use.

Literature of the time has many examples of particular new treatments and patent designs for special equipment. Each innovation would be a good marketing tool to keep ahead of the competition. By 1916, John Weber Junior was able to patent a new type of clay or terracotta couch for mud baths. The new system was heated and was also easier to clean; an important consideration in a mud or peat bath. With increasing popularity, the baths at Moor Downs grew and another wing was added in 1921. Then, in 1926, a women's bath was constructed, with a further east wing in 1928. The capacity of the treatment baths was for up to 200 visitors per day processed in 108 rooms. However, things were about to change and in 1929, following the Stock Market Crash and the Great Depression, the Grand View Health Resort moved its attention to wealthy visitors from

Chicago seeking slot machines, poker, golf, mud baths and massages. The mud-therapy market dwindled and the business was sold after the Second World War. The buildings were used as a college and are now local authority offices. Yet by the late twentieth century, there was a revival in mud and peat baths and bathing in the USA and new sites were opening to fulfil a demand. Across Europe, especially around the Baltic and the Black Sea resorts, the popularity had never waned. The interest and demand extend back almost continuously to the Roman hot spas in the Bay of Naples. The two magic ingredients were either one or both of peat and hot mud from sulphurous volcanic springs.

MIXING THE TREATMENTS AND THERAPIES

Another balance in the curative processes was that between bathing or washing in the waters and actually imbibing them. In medieval and later times, it was more common to arrive at the well-head to bathe in the waters rather than to drink them. The latter caught on only slowly until the early eighteenth century and the construction and opening of the first 'pump room'. In Roman times, with the exception of certain hot springs, it was the practice to bring the water to the baths. In most medieval curative well-heads, the water emanated into a nearby pond or pool, and the person seeking the benefits generally immersed themselves up to their necks in the spring waters. The recipient would often kneel as if in prayer or in fact actually praying. If the well or spring was smaller and more limited in volume, then the precious liquid might be applied directly to the target of the cure – such as the eyes or perhaps arthritic legs or some other part of the body. Some of the water was always drunk, and as control of and interest in the waters shifted from clerics to physicians, the practice of drinking the healing waters increased.

The whole process underwent a further change that began in European Silesia in the early 1800s. The 'water cure' was pioneered by an Austrian practitioner, Vincentz Priestnitz, who set up a hydropathic clinic and in so doing, established a whole new genre of treatment and major allegations of 'quackery'. His approach was copied and modified by hydropathic practitioners in Britain, notably Dr Wilson and Dr Gully of Malvern, John Smedley of Matlock, and Dr William MacLeod of Ben Rhydding (Ilkley) in Yorkshire. The leading lights in Britain were the first two gentlemen, Wilson and Gully, and their influence over hydropathy was enormous. The practices included extreme applications of cold water and all-over body wraps. Accusations of quackery were supported by a number of patients actually dying during treatment, though whether this was because of the treatment is a moot point; most appeared to have succumbed to heart attacks.

Bath itself had been one of the first major spa centres to move unwittingly towards hydrotherapy regimes in the later 1700s. Alongside bathing in the waters it had become the practice to 'bucket' the patrons by emptying buckets of hot spa water onto the affected body-parts requiring attention. This was soon replaced by intensive pumping of hot water onto the body, with some patients being subject to 500 'pumps' daily. Further benefits accrued from the perspiration that followed hot bathing. By the early to mid-nineteenth century the new wave of hydropathy arrived and was quickly adopted by the fashion-conscious spas.

The hydropathy treatments centred on two contrasting cold-water applications. 'Wet sheeting' involved taking the waters wrapped in wet linen sheets. The 'douche' amounted to being inundated with ice-cold water from an overhead pipe whilst sitting naked beneath it. It has to be said that the cold douche was not for the faint-hearted and the associated heart-attacks may well have been caused by this drastic treatment. This seems a far cry from the great Roman *thermae* and their luxurious and luxuriant experiences, but close to the Roman cold bath therapies. Hydropathy was intended to cure rather than to be enjoyed. Innovations included hot baths, vapour baths, hot-air baths, compressed-air baths, sweat baths or lamp-baths, with the patient covered in a heavy coarse blanket under which burnt a lamp to provide heat. A patient might lose pounds in weight in only a week. The compressed-air baths were developed by William MacLeod of Yorkshire and were highly recommended for bronchial and asthmatic patients. He also applied it to cure deafness, chronic migraine, and milder forms of tuberculosis. The owner of Lea Mill at Matlock in Derbyshire in fact underwent a remarkable conversion whilst experiencing MacLeod's rain-bath treatment of high-pressure jets of water sprayed through tiny holes in the walls of the treatment cubicle. He was at once converted to the water-cure and to Methodism; both would have a profound impact on his workforce. Fortunately though, he soon relented on the water 'douche' and observed that this cold-water treatment was primitive and 'outrageous'.

Perhaps the main reason for the apparent success of hydropathy in curing some illnesses was due to the healthy regime which accompanied the treatment. This included a modest diet, fifteen to eighteen or more Grafenburg glasses of water taken daily and energetic walking on the local hills. Removal of the patient from dirty industrial cities, smog and poor sanitation, and abstinence from tobacco, snuff, drugs, sweets, excessive drinking of alcohol, and eating only plain, simple food, probably all combined to bring about some remarkable recoveries.

The widespread Hydros, hotels offering health cures, turned away from the quackery and mystery of hydropathy during the later 1800s, and started to offer more technological treatments, especially those associated with the discoveries of electricity and radiation. These cures were to include faradisation, ergotherapy, electrotherapy, and a variety of 'pneumatic' cures. In order to keep their customers, some of these establishments broke with the no smoking rules and others even began to offer alcohol as part of the treatment. Furthermore, many of the new cures and treatments abandoned the ideas of healthy living and exercise which had probably been responsible, inadvertently, for many of the tangible benefits of the old hydrotherapy. Increasing attacks from the medical profession and damning articles in the medical journal *The Lancet* contributed to the rapid fall from grace. However, other social changes were taking their toll as well. People were generally under more pressure for time and work, and they simply didn't have time for the complicated and often long-term spa treatments. In the past, a patron might attend a clinic or spa for weeks on end, and then perhaps move on to another one for a different part of the cure. By the early twentieth century, the spa visitor expected a cure within a few days of starting the treatment; this was never going to be the case.

As straight-forward water treatment went out of fashion, it was supplanted by new technical innovations. Electrotherapy involved the patient having electric current passed through them whilst in a bath or hot water, or in some cases if required, hot peat. This could even be combined with a rectal or vaginal douche. The treatment was claimed to be good for rheumatism, for arthritis, and for gastric complaints. Various forms of electrotherapy were on offer with slightly different takes on the theme. Galvanism was the passing of an electric current through the patient's body with an attendant-cum-electrician administering the treatment. The attendant was instructed to first of all pass the dosage through him or herself, to check that it was at the right level! The effects of this process were supposedly the toning up of the body and especially the nervous system. Faradisation had a number of variants but the basic approach was for the patient to sit with their feet against a large electrode whilst the other end of the circuit was attached to the different target parts of the body.

Alongside the electric treatments the larger Hydros also had Inhalatoria which, as the name implies involved inhalation. The idea that underpinned this approach was that the vapours effectively bypassed customary drug treatments given orally, in that they did not rely on an over-strained stomach but went straight to the seat of the problem. The prescribed active substances were the types of treatments used in any inhalation process and probably worked to a degree. Apparently the Inhalatoria were especially frequented by those with laryngitis and who used their voices in their professions, such as singers, actors and of course clerics.

However, the final step away from the medieval origins – and the longer time-line back to Roman and Greek times – was another technological or at least scientific innovation that for a short time became hugely popular. The treatment was with the newly discovered radiation and two chemical elements: Radium (Ra) and Radon (Rn). The former is a heavy metal and is a million times more radioactive than the equivalent mass of Uranium. The latter is one of the so-called inert gases and one of the few gases to be intensely radioactive. Radioactivity was being discovered and understood in the late 1800s and early 1900s, and its active principles, the radioactive elements, were received as miracle cures for all sorts of ailments. This was before people working with radioactive substances began to die. It was quickly realised that these were especially dangerous substances. Yet even today, the treatment of casual ailments by exposure to radiation, albeit to smaller amounts, remains in use. Targeted medicinal applications of high-level dosages of specific radiation sources are very important in the treatment of some cancers.

High concentrations of Radon can be found in some spring waters and hot springs such as at Boulder, Montana, USA and Bad Kreuznach, Germany. To be classified as a Radon mineral water the Radon concentration must be higher than nCi/L (74 kBq/m^3). The activity of Radon mineral water in Italy reaches 2,000 kBq/m^3 in Merano, and 4,000 kBq/m^3 in Lurisia. Radioactive water baths have been in use in Jáchymov in the Czech Republic since 1906. Prior to the discovery of Radon they were used in Bad Gastein in Austria. Spas featuring Radium-rich water are still sometimes promoted as health-giving, and so Radium-rich springs which emit Radon are used in the traditional Japanese '*onsen*' in Misasa in the Tottori Prefecture. They are also used for drinking therapy at Bad Brambach in Germany. There is also inhalation therapy at Gasteiner-Heilstollen in Austria, at Świeradów-Zdrój, Czerniawa-Zdrój, Kowary and Lądek Zdrój in Poland, at Harghita Băi in Romania, and Boulder in the United States. Furthermore, in both the United States and Europe there are several 'Radon spas' where patients sit for minutes or even hours in a high-Radon atmosphere. This is in the belief that low doses of radiation will invigorate or energise them. Because of its supposed curative powers, Radium was even an additive to products like toothpaste, hair cream, and food. Once the dangers of radiation toxicity and carcinogenicity became known, these products fell from fashion and most were banned. In the United States, from the late 1940s through the early 1970s, nasal Radium irradiation was given to children to prevent middle-ear problems or enlarged tonsils.

Many spas tried to market themselves to a gullible public by association with the latest fad of radiation. Even Bath and Buxton, long-established, upmarket spa-towns, claimed their waters to be richly endowed with health-giving radiation. It was suggested that this substance, which was not applied directly to the patients, was simply in the airs and waters of these healthy resorts. Even today however, there are still so-called 'health mines' such as in Basin, Montana (USA) where people wanting relief from illnesses like arthritis go in order to receive exposure to the radioactive mine-water and to gaseous Radon. This is despite the well-documented risks to miners through long-term exposure in such situations. It is surprising what people will believe or endure in the search for a cure.

9

THE BATHS TODAY

In the post-Second World War period, there was a general downturn in traditional spas and especially in the older more natural cures. In an age of modern technology, of medical sciences and high-pressure living, there seemed no need or space for spas. Their nature-based cures seemed rather quaint, and the technological applications really jarred with their original purpose. Yet, by the 1980s and 1990s, there was a renewed interest and enthusiasm for both alternative remedies, as medical science time and again seemed to fail to deliver on basic health care. Alongside this has been an upsurge in ideas of healthy living, of spas as places for recuperation and relaxation, and an association between fitness, gymnasia and health. The new generation of spas includes expensive holiday resorts and facilities to enable the wealthy to de-stress and detox, and local health centres offering swimming, a gymnasium, saunas and spas. The latter facilities are part of an emerging modern lifestyle choice. Here, people meet and mingle, exercise and relax, swim and perspire; all this is a part of their daily routine. Remarkably in many ways, this takes the patrons back almost to where the story began two-to-three thousand years ago in Greece and in Rome. These modern-day facilities provide exactly the same type of experience that was part of the daily routine of a Romano-British citizen in Aquae Sulis in the early part of the first millennium. We even have the less salubrious 'saunas and massage parlours' operating under the broad disguise of health facilities just as the Romans did. It appears that some things never change.

With the new interest in spas and baths in the eighteenth and nineteenth centuries, the ancient sites were revisited, their waters re-examined and the buildings either restored or built anew. Then again, there followed a period of decline through the middle part of the twentieth century and a revival in the later decades. This chapter examines what is left of the numerous spas, watering places and healing baths, and particularly, of the once great bathhouses of the Romans in Britain. A list of some of the main sites, especially those which can be visited, was given in Chapter 5.

Many sites have been totally destroyed or lost, and numerous smaller baths and bathhouses from Romano-British times must remain as ruins to be rediscovered at some future date. So deeply embedded was this part of Roman culture and living that every major Roman town or fort would have had its bathhouse. Wells and springs were also very significant and many sites still remain dotted across the British landscape. Some pre-date their Roman attachments, and those which survived in medieval times were adopted by the Christian Church and given Christian saints. These wells and springs often continued up to modern times as healing sites and curative waters. Generally, where significant sites survived and were known in the twentieth century, they were accorded a degree of protection. Certainly in the post-1950s period, local authorities, charitable conservation bodies like the National Trust(s), and agencies such as English Heritage and its equivalents in Scotland and Wales, have often stepped in to conserve and manage sites and ruins.

The inventory in Chapter 5 gives some details of sites which can be visited, and these range from limited ruins of once-minor baths to monuments remaining from formerly magnificent bathhouses. Cities like York have remarkable Roman baths now preserved as a museum under the rooms of a public house, and Caerleon in South Wales has a wonderful museum to demonstrate how a major military bathhouse looked and functioned. To visit these sites and their facilities is almost to walk back into a long-forgotten era.

However, the most remarkable British site is at Bath itself. Here we have the nearest thing to a degree of continuity with Romano-British bathing. Probably deserted for a while during the early times of the Saxon invasion, there is much which remains intact at Bath in both the physical entity of the bathhouses and also in the culture of bathing.

Other major spa towns still thriving today include the grand Georgian creations such as Harrogate, Tunbridge Wells, and Cheltenham Spa, and these mix tourism, conferencing, and a quiet sense of self-contented affluence. However, of the great spa centres, other than Bath, only Buxton has a real connection to Roman bathing. In Buxton it is suggested that the modern-day Natural Baths have been used as an important water supply, a Romano-British votive (religious gift) site, and a place for bathing, for over two thousand years. A victim of the twentieth century decline in spa visiting, and ravaged by both the 1940s war effort and the burgeoning National Health Service, Buxton's traditional spa facilities suffered badly. In 1960, the Natural Baths became the town's swimming pool but this closed in 1972. However, despite the trials and tribulations of recent decades, Buxton's famous thermal mineral waters continue to be drawn from the spring for bottling. The now well-known mineral water brand, part of Nestlé's global bottled water operation, provides a link back to the Roman legionnaires who visited or settled at Buxton to take the waters and to bathe here.

The town has had major investment in recent decades to repair and reinstate the grand buildings. Perhaps some of the future works may expose and be able to celebrate the Roman origins of Buxton which so far have proved tantalisingly difficult to find. Perhaps they do lie under the former St Ann's Hotel at the western end of the Crescent. This hotel stayed open until 1989 when the serving of public health notices for dirty kitchens forced its closure. The then-owners were unwilling or unable to finance the costly repairs that were needed, and by 1993 it was in such a poor state of repair that, in a landmark case, the Department of National Heritage served a legal notice threatening compulsory purchase. Consequently, the owners were forced to agree a sale, funded by a grant from the National Heritage Memorial Fund, to the High Peak Borough Council. The latter took on a role of caretaker owner until a longer-term strategy was in place. An additional English Heritage grant of £1.5 million was made available for essential structural repairs. Perhaps one day the full story of Buxton's Roman past will be revealed and told.

10

THE CITY OF BATH

THESE
HEALING WATERS
HAVE FLOWED ON
FROM TIME UNDATED
TO THIS DAY.
THEIR VIRUE UNIMPAIRED
THEIR VOLUME UNABATED
THER HEAT UNDIMINISHED
THEY EXPLAIN
THE ORIGIN,
ACCOUNT FOR THE PROGRESS,
AND DEMAND THE GRATITUDE
OF THE CITY OF BATH

– Statement from a plaque in the city of Bath

BATH AND THE WATERS

Bath is a unique place in Britain and is special in both European and global terms as a hot-water spa. The city owes its justifiable fame to a geological fault running deep into the volcanic core of the Earth. Research has confirmed that the 'Waters' emanate from rocks around two miles below Bath. The passage of water takes around 10,000 years from the surface and into deep bedrocks below the Bristol and Radstock coalfields, where it begins the slow rise at a temperature of 70°C to reach the surface at about 45°C and to make Bath the only truly 'hot' spring in Britain. Around 1 million litres or about 250,000 gallons of low-concentration mineral water emerge each day and this is the basis of the economy and the reputation of the city. The reduced levels of mineral salts make the water good for flushing out the kidneys, and at one time, the occurrence of low-level background radiation was also seen as health-giving. Bath has enjoyed three golden periods in its history: the Roman times, the eighteenth-century revival, and a modern renaissance.

THE EMERGENCE OF THE MODERN CITY

Modern Bath is a major tourist destination and its Roman baths remain at core of its reputation. Furthermore, the recent investment in major refurbishment has placed Bath back once again in its position as the leading global attraction for a unique bathing experience. This bathing extravaganza takes the visitor back nearly two thousand years to the glory days of the Roman Empire. Modern Bath is a city located 97 miles (156 km) west of London and 13 miles (21 km) south-east of Bristol, in the old English county of Somerset. Granted city status by Royal Charter by Queen Elizabeth I in 1590, today it has a population of a little over 80,000 residents and many visiting tourists. It became a County Borough in 1889, a move that provided administrative independence from its parent county of Somerset. Having become a part of the newly created county of Avon in 1974, since 1996, when that county was abolished, Bath has taken responsibility as the main administrative centre of the Unitary Authority of 'Bath and North East Somerset'. In 1987, the City of Bath was designated a World Heritage Site and it now boasts numerous theatres, museums, and other cultural and sporting venues. Together these facilities and the unique historic context help make Bath a major tourism centre. It has over a million staying visitors and 3.8 million day-visitors each year. There are also two universities and several schools and colleges. The modern city has a large service sector, expanding information and communication technologies, and developing creative industries. All these provide employment for the people of Bath itself but also for the surrounding areas. The Bath Hospital, now the Royal National Hospital for Rheumatic Diseases, was established in 1742 and has long been the leading centre for the treatment of rheumatism and rehabilitation.

A WATERING PLACE WITH A LONG HISTORY

The city has a long history and a rich lineage with continuity from ancient times to the modern world. For example, the hills around Bath such as

Bathampton Down have abundant evidence of human occupation and activity from the Middle Stone Age or Mesolithic Period onwards. Later activity is evidence by a number of Bronze Age round barrows which were opened by John Skinner in the eighteenth century. The prehistoric structure of Bathampton Camp was probably an Iron Age hill-fort or stock enclosure, and a 'long barrow' site, believed to be from the Beaker people *c.* 2400–1800 BC (late Neolithic to Bronze Ages), and was demolished to construct RAF Charmy Down. Evidence of settlement on the higher ground, well away from the valley-bottom wetlands, comes from finds like the gold-plated sun disc dating back to around 1600 BC found at a barrow on Lansdown.

IRON AGE AND ROMAN BEGINNINGS

Ptolemy, writing in Roman Egypt in the second century AD, described the Roman buildings at Bath as one of the wonders of the world; a remarkable transformation from what, only shortly before this time, was a boggy pool in a great marsh. The town of Bath was first established by the Romans in AD 43, as a spa bearing the Roman Latin name of Aquae Sulis ('The Waters of Sulis'), but this was already a sacred site for the local Celts. The Fosseway, running north-south, crossed the River Avon by two fords, one of which was located where the weir is today. Following the discovery of the hot spring the Romans built baths, a water supply reservoir and a large temple on the hills surrounding Bath and in the valley of the River Avon. The Roman developments were centred on and around the hot springs. The most significant structure remaining from this work is the Great Bath at the Roman Baths, though the entire structure above the level of the pillar bases is a more modern reconstruction. The archaeological evidence shows that the site of the main spring for the Roman Baths was a religious shrine used by the Celtic Iron Age Britons, and was dedicated to their goddess Sulis. The Romans identified her with their own deity, Minerva. Messages to her scratched onto metal, known as curse tablets, have been found by archaeologists at the site of the bathhouse. These curse tablets were written in Latin and placed a curse on those who in the eyes of the writer had done them wrong. For example, if a patron had his clothes or other belongings stolen at the baths, he could write a curse. This would name the suspects if known, on a tablet to be read by the Goddess Sulis Minerva. One, written backwards as to be only read by a god or goddess, cursed 'he who carried off Vilbia' presumably someone's wife or girlfriend.

The temple, measuring 66 feet by 33 feet, was constructed from around AD 60–70 and the bathhouse complex was gradually developed over the following three centuries. During the Roman occupation of Britain and perhaps under instruction from Emperor Claudius or his advisors, engineers drove oaken piles into the mud of the site where the spring emanated to provide a stable foundation. The spring was then surrounded by an irregular stone chamber lined with lead. Later, in the second century, the spring was further enclosed within a barrel-vaulted wooden building. This structure housed the *calidarium* (hot bath), the *tepidarium* (warm bath), and the *frigidarium* (cold bath). The temple had Corinthian columns with a pediment, on the centre of which was a statue of a Gorgon's head, now a choice exhibit in the modern museum. Also in the temple area was an altar with four carved corner-stones, three of which are on display. On the base-stone is inscribed: 'To the Goddess Sul, Lucious Marcius aruspex', the last word meaning 'augurer', or one who foretells the future by examining the entrails of ritually slaughtered animals. Many of the finds on display at Bath are from offerings or gifts to the Goddess thrown into the spring. They include a collection of thirteen pewter vessels and many minor trinkets. Much of the Roman 'archaeology' sank back into the swamp after the collapse of the Roman Empire and, like the gilt-bronze head of Minerva and a set of carved gemstones, was not rediscovered until the eighteenth or nineteenth centuries.

As a major and important centre for Romano-British activities, the city had defensive walls built around it in about the third century. However, these defences couldn't make up for the wider collapse of the Roman Empire and the rapid withdrawal of troops to Italy itself. After the abandonment of Britain in the early years of the fifth century, Aquae Sulis and its baths fell rapidly into disrepair. The baths themselves, and their contents, were eventually lost back into the mire and silts from which they had been born.

BROKEN AND RUINED: POST-ROMAN AND MEDIEVAL TIMES

As the Romans left Britain Bath soon fell into disrepair, and the ruins soon either sank back into the swamp or were simply over-topped by mud, silt and peat as nature reasserted itself. At this time few could have imagined that over the following thousand years or so, Bath would once again rise from the wetlands that gave it life.

The precise history of Bath in post-Roman times is not always clear, and like many early settlements it has been associated with numerous historically significant events but not always with much evidence. For example, it has been suggested that Bath was the site of the Battle of Mons Badonicus (*c.* AD 500), at which King Arthur is said to have defeated the invading Anglo-Saxons. Like much of the Arthurian legend, part history and part myth, this is disputed by some authorities. However, it is known that the city fell to the West Saxons in AD 577 after the Battle of Deorham or Dyrham, and an Anglo-Saxon poem, 'The Ruin', may describe the Roman site of Bath at this time. It became a part of the Saxon kingdom of Mercia, and the broken statues of the two Saxon kings, Osric and Offa, have long stood above the entrance of No. 8 Bath Street. In the period after the fall to the Saxons, by around AD 675–76, a monastery was established maybe by Saint David but more likely by King Osric of the Hwicce, and a small bathing facility was established. The still-walled part of the old town may have been the monastic precinct. The town was renamed Ackmancaestor or Sick Man's Town. Nennius, a ninth-century historian, notes what he describes as a 'Hot Lake' in the land of the Hwicce along the River Severn. Usefully he states that 'it is surrounded by a wall, made of brick and stone, and men may go there to bathe at any time, and every man can have the kind of bath he likes. If he wants, it will be a cold bath; and if he wants a hot bath, it will be hot'. There is a similar description in the historical writings of Bede's *Ecclesiastical History*. In AD 781, King Offa of Mercia took control of the monastery and rebuilt the church, now dedicated to St Peter.

In the ninth century, now under the control of King Alfred, the old street pattern of the Roman town had gone. As a royal possession of Alfred, the town was rebuilt and laid out anew; now with the south-eastern quadrant as the abbey precinct. In the Burghal Hidage (an Anglo-Saxon document giving a list of the fortified burghs in Wessex and elsewhere in southern England), Bath is noted as possessing walls of 1,375 yards (1,257 metres) and had 1,000 men for purposes of defence. During the time of King Edward the Elder (born *c.* 874–77, died 924), coins were minted in the town. By the tenth century the place was called Bader, and then renamed Bath. Edward became king in AD 899 following the death of his father Alfred, and the coins minted at Bath were based on a design from the Winchester Mint but with 'BAD' on the obverse. This derived from the Anglo-Saxon name for the town, Baðum, Baðan or Baðon, meaning simply 'at the baths'. In AD 957, the fourteen-year-old Edgar – later known as Edgar the Peaceful – was crowned at Bath Abbey and became King of England north of the Thames, and two years later acquired the overlordship of the whole country; England was united for the first time under a single monarch. The event is commemorated in a stained glass window in the Abbey, and the name has remained as Bath ever since. The market town was gradually growing and establishing its importance but mainly as an ecclesiastical centre, the nunnery replaced by a Benedictine monastery and the waters controlled by the church.

King William II (or William Rufus) granted the town to John de Tours (or John de Villula), his royal physician, who became Bishop of Wells and Abbot of Bath. This followed the sacking of the town during the 1088 Rebellion which followed the death of William the Conqueror and related to the division and inheritance of lands in the Kingdom of England and the Duchy of Normandy. The civil war ran for three to six months from Easter 1088, and William was to die in suspicious circumstances in AD 1100. A policy of the Papacy at the time was for Bishops to move to more urban seats. In this case, John de Tours moved from Wells to Bath, and planned and designed a much enlarged church as his cathedral with a priory and bishop's palace. He also had new baths built around the three springs, but later bishops returned the episcopal seat to Wells. These later bishops retained the name of Bath in their title as the 'Bishop of Bath and Wells'. At about this time, around 1180, the St John's Hospital was founded by Bishop Reginald Fitz Jocelin; it was to become one of the oldest English almshouses. The 'hospital of the baths' was constructed close to the hot springs of the Cross Bath. This provided shelter for the poor infirm and gave them access to the health-giving waters. The cathedral was never completed and began to fall into decay and disrepair, until in the thirteenth century it was ravaged by fire.

Bath gained its first City Charter from King Richard I, largely in recognition for its support in the crusades, and the administrative title of Burgh – held since AD 577 – was changed to that of a Mayor. In fact, the process was one of selling charters to various towns and cities to grant them status and certain exemptions from taxes to encourage trade. The charters were an important means for raising much-needed revenue for the overseas war. The city today has had twenty-seven charters, and boasts a complete list of over 750 mayors since AD 1230. The administrative systems of this period were organised as so-called Hundreds, and that for Bath had a number of different names down the centuries, such as the 'Hundred of Le Buri'. The Bath 'Foreign Hundred' or *Forinsecum* covered the outside of the town but they were eventually combined as the 'Bath Forum Hundred'. Increasingly, the wealthy merchants of the town, lacking status at the 'Hundred Courts', formed guilds to organise themselves and to grow their political and social influence. The first guildhall was built sometime in the thirteenth century, and the town got its first mayor early in that same century.

A DIRTY, SMELLY CITY: EARLY MODERN BATH

By the fifteenth century, the Abbey church was in poor condition and in dire need of repair. Oliver King, then Bishop of Bath and Wells, decided to rebuild the church but on a smaller scale in 1500. The new cathedral or Abbey was completed just as Bath Priory was being dissolved (in 1539) by order of King Henry VIII. The Abbey church fell into ruinous condition before being restored as the town's parish church, and further improved and enlarged by Bishop Montague in the seventeenth century. As the Elizabethan reign progressed Bath experienced a revival as a spa centre. As a consequence, the baths were improved and the town, granted city status by Royal Charter of Queen Elizabeth I in 1590, began to attract the aristocracy to its healing waters. This second city charter was number twenty-two on the list of twenty-seven royal decrees, and along with first city charter can be seen (by appointment) at the city archives.

During the English Civil War (1642–51), the staunchly Royalist city was held and garrisoned, with seven thousand pounds spent on strengthening the fortifications. However, when the Parliamentary forces arrived, perhaps prudently, the gates were thrown open and the city surrendered. Bath then became a significant station in Somerset for the New Model Army under their regional commander, William Waller. Despite the importance to the Parliamentary forces, the city was retaken by Royalists following the Battle of Lansdowne, on 5 July 1643, which was fought on the northern outskirts of the city. With the war over and the Commonwealth imposed on the country, the next few years saw reduced interest in the spas, despised as they were by the Puritans. However, following the Restoration, the patronage of royalty and nobility alike guaranteed a vibrant and wealthy future for the city. Indeed, when the restoration of the monarchy came to pass it is said that the conduits of Bath ran with claret, and there was a procession of 400 virgins dressed in white coats and green petticoats. As Kersley (1973) points out, from a total city population of around a thousand people, this doesn't ring true.

By medieval times, Bath had become a walled town covering around twenty-four acres and about a third of its people were connected to the church and the ecclesiastical functions. The area around the city was growing in importance for the wool trade and for coal mining and stone quarrying. Other commerce included a paper mill and a brass mill. The monks constructed a weir to provide water-power for the mill and in doing this deepened the river. This necessitated the replacement of stepping stones by a ferry, close to the present-day Pulteney Bridge. The only bridge over the River Avon was located just below Holloway, and this linked to the city's south gate by a muddy track lined by the hovels of a shanty town beyond the city walls. There was also a riverside quay where fish was sold, and a market cross with a group of small dwellings, and the city's 'ducking stool' for the punishment of gossips and prostitutes.

The city itself would have been tightly constrained within the walls, the latter being medieval structures but perhaps sat on top of earlier Roman foundations. Inside this envelope would be a mix of the grander stone-built structures, such as the Abbey and associated buildings, and a messy huddle of gabled thatched cottages and houses and poorer hovels. Cheap Street, running east-west, was barely 7 feet wide and had an open sewer down the middle, and it was this vermin-infested environment that was so conducive to bubonic plague, which arrived in AD 1349. Other buildings included Prior's Bath, School and Hospital.

The small baths constructed for Osric and Offa in the seventh and eighth centuries were replaced during the sixteenth century by five new baths. This followed on from the dissolution of the monasteries and the transfer of control over the waters from the church to the city. The five new baths were the Cross Bath and the Hot Bath (both fed from a separate source called the Hetling Spring), and the Abbot's Bath, the Prior's Bath, and the King's Bath. Sluices took the used waters back down via the Monk's Mill to the river. The Hot Baths was more recently known as the Old Royal. King Henry VIII, on visiting the baths, found the King's Bath to be 'large and fair'. At this time the healing waters were being used for the treatment of gout, skin complaints, and fertility (see Chapter 8 for example). Mary of Medina, the consort of King James II, also visited Bath to resolve fertility problems and gave birth to a prince who was later to become the Young Pretender. Not everyone liked the mixed bathing arrangements, and Princess Anne of Denmark in 1613–15 encouraged the building of the Queen's Bath adjacent to the King's Bath. Charles II in 1663 was said to be the first monarch to 'take the waters', and Bath was on the way to a new golden age.

A key point was the writing of Thomas Guidott, who had been a student of chemistry and medicine at Wadham College, Oxford. He moved to Bath and set up practice there in 1668, and became interested in the curative properties of the waters. He soon wrote *A Discourse of Bathe, and the Hot Waters There*, and then in 1676, *Some Enquiries into the Nature of the Water*. This and other publications of the period began to bring the health-giving, curative properties of the hot mineral waters to the attention of a wider audience. First the aristocracy arrived, and then everyone else who could afford it. As the spa theme developed at Bath, the town was already prosperous on account of its connections with the wool-trade, mining and quarrying. However, as already described, like most provincial towns of the time, post-medieval Bath still had narrow, unpaved streets with minimal and unhealthy sanitary arrangements. Most buildings were potential fire and health risks. Moreover, if you walked the streets of the town it was wise to be armed in case of assault. Furthermore, a visitor to Bath, unless very wealthy, would probably stay at a lodging house or an inn, which might well involve sharing a bed that teemed with bed bugs, with strangers who themselves crawled with fleas, body lice and head lice. The sheer squalor of a medieval town is scarcely imaginable to us today.

By comparison, as noted earlier, Georgian taste favoured regularity and elegance; the old rambling, dirty city was swept away to be transformed into elegant and tasteful streets and squares. Several areas of the city had undergone transformation during the Stuart Period, but this increased dramatically through the Georgian times. With increasing numbers of visitors to the now thriving spa and resort town, there was an urgent and growing need for appropriate accommodation. Father and son architects, John Wood the Elder and John Wood the Younger, designed and set out new streets, buildings and squares, with identical façades to give the impression of grand scale and classical style, to match anything in Europe. The result was the greatest concentration of fine eighteenth-century architecture anywhere in the world. The city itself needed to be planned and renewed, and a newly fashionable clientèle demanded elegant and clean accommodation to buy or to rent.

Up to this time the rich and the poor, the sick and the able-bodied, all shared the precious waters. Interestingly however, in 1714, the long-standing law giving the poor people free access to the healing waters was repealed. As a consequence, moves were made to develop the Bath Hospital to give free treatment to 150 patients 'from without the city'. It was not until 1742 that the new establishment was opened.

Combe Down and Bathampton Down limestone mines were owned by entrepreneur Ralph Allen (1694–1764), and supplied most of the beautiful creamy-gold 'Bath Stone' used for construction throughout the city. In fact this stone had already been recognised and highly valued by the Romans for their constructions, and during the seventeenth century, small quarries were once again opened. Major quarries were developed in the eighteenth century to produce the Bath Stone employed in the massive building work in Bath itself, and increasingly elsewhere in Britain, at locations including Buckingham Palace. The stone was extracted, quarried or mined by the 'room and pillar' method using chambers cut to leave pillars of stone supporting the roof. Allen was clearly onto what we might describe as a nice earner with the ownership of his quarries, and as former Postmaster General, had an eye for business. In order to advertise the good quality of his quarried limestone, he commissioned the elder John Wood to build a country house on Prior Park, his estate between the city and the mines. However, Allen was a civic-minded man to whom Bath owes a great debt and served as a member of the Bath Corporation for many years, and at the age of fifty, served one term as Mayor in 1742.

In the early eighteenth century, Bath gained its first purpose-built theatre, the Old Orchard Street Theatre. This was later rebuilt as the Theatre Royal, and with the Grand Pump Room attached to the Roman Baths, and the Assembly Rooms, provides a basis for the social and cultural life of the city. The Master of Ceremonies, Richard 'Beau' Nash, presided over the city's social life and etiquette from 1705 until his death in 1761 and drew up the famous code of behaviour for public entertainments in the city (see Chapter 8). Essentially the four men, Nash, Allen, and the Woods, were responsible for the dramatic upturn in Bath's fortunes and a threefold increase in its population. Visitors flocked to Bath because of the waters but also because it became a Mecca for the English social season. The city was described by Christopher Hussey (in Kelsey, 1973): 'A fair city that looks as if it has been cast in a mould all at once and turned out perfectly fresh and youthful'; a far cry indeed from the squalid medieval city of pickpockets and vermin.

A FINE, ELEGANT AND THRIVING CITY: LATE MODERN BATH

The population of the city had reached 40,020 by the time of the 1801 census, making it one of the largest cities in Britain, and certainly the most fashionable. With its thriving resident population and the inundation of rich socialites during the season, Bath was enormously successful and popular during this time. Patronage by famous writers and others ensured the lasting appeal of the transformed city. Like many such places with the rich and eccentric residents and patrons, Bath has a legacy of buildings and structures to reflect its colourful past, and some left a legacy of beautiful open spaces too. William Beckford for example, bought a house in Lansdown Crescent in 1822, eventually buying a further two houses in the crescent to form his residence. Having acquired all the land between his home and the top of Lansdown Hill, he created a garden over half a mile in length and built Beckford's Tower at the top. Beckford's Tower, originally known as Lansdown Tower, is an architectural folly built in the neoclassical style. Standing 120 feet (37 metres) high, the tower was completed in 1827 for Beckford to a design by Henry Goodridge. Beckford wished it had been built 40 feet higher, but remarked that 'such as it is, it is a famous landmark for drunken farmers on their way home from market'. Beckford used the tower as a library and a retreat. It is located at the end of the pleasure gardens called Beckford's Ride which ran from his house in Lansdown Crescent up to the Tower at the top of Lansdown Hill. Another famous resident, though much later and by force rather than by choice, was at Fairfield House, in Newbridge during the late 1930s. This was the official residence of His Imperial Majesty, Haile Selassie I, Emperor of Ethiopia, during the five years he spent in exile from 1936 to 1941. Following his return to Ethiopia in 1958, he donated the house to the city of Bath as a residence for the aged.

The list of famous visitors is almost endless but includes the diarist Samuel Pepys and the writer Jane Austen. Pepys describes how, at 4 a.m., he was carried to the Cross Bath for a two-hour session of being pumped at two pence per hundred strokes, or bucketed. During the latter he notes that he was given a crownless hat to wear; men generally wore a coat and drawers and ladies a canvas cover. Following their bath, the visitors would be carried back to bed in a sedan chair, something which necessitates particularly wide turning on many stairways in the city. The waters would be 'taken' or drunk three times a day and this was considered excellent therapy for gout, for example. When important visitors arrived at the city the town bells were pealed and a Town Crier announced their names. Pope, Defoe, Smollett, Herschel, Dickens, Coleridge, Horace Walpole, Clive of India, Wolfe of Quebec, Sheridan, Siddons, William Pitt and Irving, are just some of the great and famous visitors and residents who spent time at the city.

In the eighteenth century, a visit to the baths would also very often be followed by one to the gaming rooms and the dance halls – Harrisons, Wiltshires, and Gydes – and then later to the assembly rooms. However, in 1745, gambling was made illegal and this lucrative but highly risky trade was curtailed. Bath continued to be a favourite place to visit through the Victorian period, though its fortunes, so closely tied to 'the waters', were to ebb and flow as did the fashions for bathing in and drinking spa water. During the 1800s, the interest in sulphur-rich waters emerged and, despite efforts to prove otherwise, Bath-water was low in this mineral. However, claims to low background radiation levels and so associated curative properties were still being made in the early 1900s to boost the falling appeal of spa bathing.

Anstey, writing the *New Bath Guide*, in 1766, described the experience over the period of the late eighteenth and early nineteenth centuries:

> T'was a glorious sight to behold the fair sex
> All wading with gentlemen up to their necks
> And today Many persons of rank and condition
> Were boiled by command of an able physician!

THROUGH THE NINETEENTH AND TWENTIETH CENTURIES: A SLOW DECLINE AND A RAPID REBIRTH

Bath, in the twenty-first century, is clearly in a third golden age as a modern tourism city with a global reputation. However, this evolution has not always been easy, nor indeed predicable. Looking back, whilst the Georgian revolution in Bath's architecture was dramatic and spectacular, clearly much was removed that we would now value highly in terms of medieval architecture and features. It is a shame that more was not salvaged and incorporated into the newly reborn city, but that is merely a modern-day reflective view. The city was bursting with people and the building of the new required the destruction and removal of the old. Sadly, the old city walls were demolished and the walks near the Abbey destroyed. The old Guildhall, perhaps designed by Inigo Jones, was demolished as it was felt to be a traffic hazard. Union Street was built, and to put the destruction into perspective, the compensation for loss of buildings amounted to about £30,000; for the time a colossal sum. The Bear Inn, reputed to be one of the finest hostelries in the kingdom, was a casualty, as too was the White Hart. The Saracen's Head, built in 1713 and still standing today, was where Charles Dickens wrote *The Pickwick Papers*. During this architectural whirlwind, the city also lost two-thirds of its old churches. In the 1800s the Circus gained its Plane Trees, adding greenery and shade but also issues of management and of overshadowing buildings. Most of the houses were owned privately, often by doctors who resided and consulted in their home. In the Royal Crescent, a household would employ four to eight maids who each had one day off per week, and had to be in by nine o'clock in the evening. On an income of, say, £1,000 you could easily employ three maids, a cook, a coachman, and a footman. Ordinary people travelled the city by tram as, for example, for only three old pence you could get from Combe Down to Bathford. The city thrived even though the pattern of bathing and water cures changed as described earlier. Up to the Second World War, Bath still had four hotels with five-star classification: The Pump Room, The Pulteney, the Empire and the Spa.

Even the water supply was to change over this period. Whereas it had long been from the plentiful local springs, by the mid-nineteenth century it was managed by the Corporation with centralised supply, storage, treatment and distribution. By 1818 the city had town gas, and by 1890, electricity. There was a canal and the railways were to follow.

With its history and development over the centuries so closely linked to medicine and healing, it is hardly surprising that Bath boasts a long list of eminent and influential physicians. This roll-call of honour includes seven Fellows of the Royal Society, one being Caleb Hillier Parry, a contemporary of Edward Jenner. His work was particularly important in understanding and treating thyro-toxicosis and angina. William Oliver FRS, as well as being a physician of renown, invented the recipe for the famous Bath Oliver Biscuit. By the twentieth century however, much of the rationale behind the success of the Bath waters was in decline. The quackery that had crept into hydrotherapy treatments and the like was rife, and there was even a rigorous, authoritarian separation of male and female patients during treatment. All this was a far cry from the heyday of visiting Bath to take the waters. By the 1930s, moves were afoot to place the health treatments on a more rigorous scientific basis and to concentrate particularly on issues of arthritis and rheumatism. This is the foundation for the modern-day reputation of the Bath hospitals, and despite major policy and funding battles with the Health Service in the 1950s the specialist centres in rheumatology now have a worldwide reputation. Further impetus to this development was the establishment and growth of the University of Bath in the 1970s.

Bath is still a city of surprises. Aside from its early history in civil wars and earlier invasions, one would imagine twentieth-century Bath to be an unlikely target for enemy aggression. However, during the Second World War, from the evening of 25 April to the early morning of 27 April 1942, Bath suffered three major air raids. These were in reprisal for RAF raids on the German cities of Lübeck and Rostock, and were a part of the Luftwaffe campaign known as the 'Baedeker Blitz'. The Baedeker Blitz or Baedeker raids were a series of *Vergeltungsangriffe* ('retaliatory raids') by the German air force on English cities. This was a direct response to the bombing of the Hanseatic League City of Lübeck during the night 28/29 March 1942. Arthur 'Bomber' Harris, Air Officer Commanding RAF Bomber Command, wrote of the raid that 'Lübeck went up in flames' because 'it was a city of moderate size of some importance as a port, and with some submarine building yards of moderate size not far from it. It was not a vital target, but it seemed to me better to destroy an industrial town of moderate importance than to fail to destroy a large industrial city'. The Area Bombing Directive issued to the RAF on 14 February 1942 focused on the 'morale of the enemy civil population'. Lübeck, with its numerous medieval timbered buildings, was chosen because the RAF 'Air Staff were eager to experiment with a bombing technique using a high proportion of incendiaries' to help them carry out the directive.

Because cities like Coventry had been subject to such Luftwaffe attacks during the Blitz, the RAF were well aware that this technique was effective against cities but not necessarily against major industrial targets. In retaliation for the Lübeck raid, the Germans bombed Exeter on 23 April 1942, the first of the 'Baedeker' raids. The Lübeck raid along with that on Rostock caused 'outrage in the German leadership ... and inspired the retaliatory "Baedeker" raids'. In Bath, over 400 people were killed, and more than 19,000 buildings were damaged or destroyed. Houses in the Royal Crescent, the Circus and the Paragon were burnt out. This loss was along with the Assembly Rooms, and part of the south side of Queen Square; a shocking and surprising part of the city's history.

Like in many English post-war cities, the impact of the Blitz went beyond the mere damage from the bombers. The 1950s city planners finished off much that the bombers failed to achieve. A post-war review of poor inner-city housing led to the clearance and redevelopment of slum areas of the city in a typical post-war modern style. The 1960s rebuilding caused irrevocable and unforgivable damage to much of the earlier heritage. This change was often at variance with the local Georgian style which by now was often considered outdated and passé. In the 1950s, the nearby villages of Combe Down, Twerton and Weston were also incorporated into Bath to enable the development of further housing, much of it Council Housing. The urban sprawl typical of so many towns was underway.

However, during the 1970s and 1980s, there was a gradual recognition of the damage that was being done, and also of the severe problems of traffic congestion and associated pollution. It was understood that the conservation of Bath's historic buildings was inadequate and that much damage had been done and many unique structures lost or compromised. This led to more care and the reuse and restoration of buildings and open spaces. In 1987, in recognition of its unique international cultural significance, the city was selected by UNESCO as a World Heritage Site. Spurred on by this success and the enhanced status, since 2000, developments have included the Bath Spa, South Gate and the Bath Western Riverside project. The city is now both thoroughly modern but also, for the most part, wonderfully preserved. From before the Romans, the City of Bath had emerged from the great swamps of the Avon valley to develop as a grand city only to sink back into the mire. Then, phoenix-like, it had risen again and gradually decayed only to be rebuilt afresh. Today, as one of the most beautiful cities in the world, albeit with a sometimes chequered history, Bath is well into a third golden age and its thermal waters still attract visitors from far and wide.

Kelsey (1973) ends his little book, *Bath Water*, with a nice – albeit slightly erroneous – quote about the healing waters, and here I give the corrected version. Lorenz Fries, a writer of popular medical books in the sixteenth century, stated in his *Spiegel der Artzny* (1518) a series of treatments for painful joints: 'Roast a fat old goose and stuff with chopped kittens, lard, incense, wax and the flour of rye. This must all be eaten and the drippings applied to the painful joints ... It then withdraws the pains in the joints.' He also advocates that 'the sodden flesh of a weasel or cat, tied over the rheumatic joint, allays the pain'; as does 'the fat of a fox well rubbed in', or 'a warm and bleeding pigeon applied to the soles of the feet'. The point is that, as noted by cynics, the 'Waters' are one of the few medical 'cures' that never did anyone any harm. Furthermore, some of the treatments advocated in earlier times are less than inviting, whereas the 'Waters', even if not always effective, were often delightful!

BIBLIOGRAPHY

Alderson, F. (1973) *The Inland Resorts and Spas of Britain*. David & Charles, Newton Abbot, Devon.

Anon. (undated) *The Spas of Britain: The Official Handbook of the British Spa Federation*. Pitman Press, Bath.

Anon. (undated) *A pictorial and descriptive guide to Bath, Cheddar, Wells, Glastonbury, etc.* Tenth edition, Ward, Lock & Co. Ltd, London.

Anon. (2004) *Spa Style Europe: Therapies, Cuisines, Spas*. Weatherhill, New York.

Ashenburg, K. (2007) *CLEAN: The Unsanitized History of Washing*. Profile Books, London.

Ball, P. (1999) *H_2O: A Biography of Water*. Weidenfeld & Nicholson, London.

Cunliffe, B. (1980) The excavation of the Roman Spring at Bath 1979. A preliminary description. *The Antiquaries Journal*, LX (II), 187–206.

Eyre, H. (1733) *An Account of the Mineral Waters of SPA, Commonly called the German SPAW: being a collection of observations from the most Eminent Authors who have wrote on that Subject*. J. Roberts, Warwick Lane, London.

Fagan, G. G. (1999) Bathing in Public in the Roman World. The University of Michegan Press, Ann Arbor, USA.

Frere, S. (1967) *Britannia: A History of Roman Britain*. Routledge & Kegan Paul Ltd, London.

Granville, A. B. (1841) *Spas of England and principal sea-bathing places. 1: the North*. Reprinted in 1971 by Adams & Dart, Bath.

Granville, A. B. (1841) *Spas of England and principal sea-bathing places. 2: the Midlands and South*. Reprinted in 1971 by Adams & Dart, Bath.

Havins, P. J. N. (1976) *The Spas of England*. Robert Hale & Company, London.

Hibbert, C. (1985) *Rome: The Biography of a City*. Viking-Penguin Books Ltd., Harmondsworth, UK.

Jones, W. H. S. & Ross, R. (1907) *Malaria: A neglected Factor in the History of Greece and Rome*. Macmillan & Co. Ltd, London.

Kersley, G. D. (1973) *Bath Water: The Effects of the Waters on the History of Bath and of Medicine*. Victor Morgan Books Ltd, Bath. (Revised edition published in 1979 by Bath City Council, Bath).

Langham, M. & Wells, C. (1986) *Buxton Waters: A History of Buxton the Spa*. J. H. Hall & Sons Ltd., Derby.

Langham, M. & Wells, C. (1997) *A History of the Baths at Buxton*. Churnet Valley Books, Leek, Staffordshire.

Laurence, R. (2009) *Roman Passions: A History of Pleasure in Imperial Rome*. Continum, London.

Lomas, P. (2007) *The Buxton Hydro (Spa Hotel): The Story of the Spa Town's best known Hydropathic between 1866 and 1974*. Country Books/ Ashridge Press, Bakewell.

Newton, B. (1989) *Ravenglass through the Ages*. British Nuclear Fuels plc, Sellafield, Cumbria.

Rolf, V. (2011) *Bathing Houses and Plunge Pools*. Shire Publications, Oxford.

Rook, T. (1976) A visit to the Welwyn Roman baths is a memorable experience. *Hertfordshire Countryside*, 31 (205), May 1976, 32–33.

Rook, T. (1992; second edition 2002) *Roman Baths in Britain*. Shire Archaeology, Risborough, Buckinghamshire.

Rosen, W. (2007) *Justinian's flea: Plague, Empire and the Birth of Europe*. Viking-Penguin Books Ltd., London.

Searle, M. (1977) *Spas and Watering Places*. MIDAS Books, Tunbridge Wells, Kent.

Smith, V. (2007) *CLEAN: A History of Personal Hygiene and Purity*. Oxford University Press, Oxford.

Wilson, R. (1980) *Roman Forts: An Illustrated Introduction to the Garrison Posts of Roman Britain*. Bergstrom & Boyle books Limited, London.

Yegül, F. (2010) *Bathing in the Roman World*. Cambridge University Press, Cambridge.

INDEX

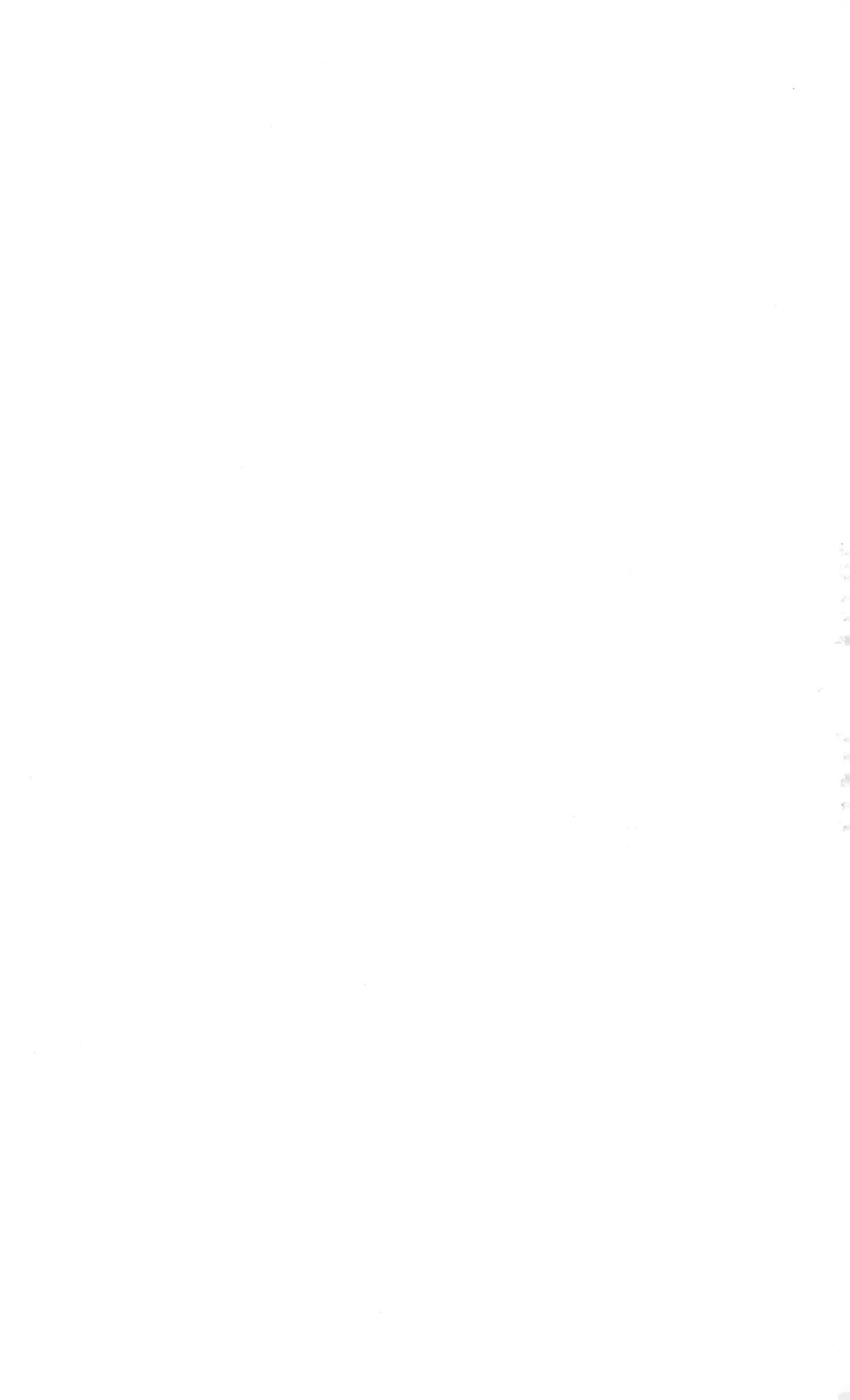